Crowdsourcing during COVID-19

Crowdsourcing is a means by which public interest is sought and leveraged to achieve specific goals, and this fascinating study highlights how the model has been used to challenge the effects of the COVID-19 pandemic.

The book investigates what factors have encouraged the use of crowdsourcing during the pandemic, as well as those issues which have restricted its use. It is illustrated with four detailed case studies, covering the fields of education and health, demonstrating how crowdsourcing as a means of crisis management has, ultimately, been used to influence and develop public policy.

A timely analysis of this emerging concept, the book will appeal to researchers and practitioners across health and social care, public policy and management, and the voluntary sector more generally.

Carmen Bueno Muñoz is a student of the PhD program in economics and business at the University of Extremadura (Spain). Her research interests are the digital transformation of the economy and innovation.

Luis R. Murillo Zamorano is the director of the Research Group in Economic Analysis and Marketing Management (AEDIMARK R&D Group) at the University of Extremadura and is an associate professor in the Department of Economics at the University of Extremadura, Spain.

José Ángel López Sánchez has a PhD degree from the University of Oviedo (Spain), is a researcher in the Research Group on Economic Analysis and Marketing Management (AEDIMARK R&D Group) at the University of Extremadura (Spain), and is an associate professor in the marketing and market research area at the University of Extremadura (Spain).

Crowdsourcing during COVID-19

Case Studies in Health and Education

Carmen Bueno Muñoz, Luis R. Murillo Zamorano and José Ángel López Sánchez

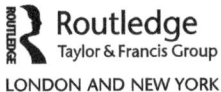
Routledge
Taylor & Francis Group

LONDON AND NEW YORK

First published 2022
by Routledge
2 Park Square, Milton Park, Abingdon, Oxon OX14 4RN

and by Routledge
605 Third Avenue, New York, NY 10158

Routledge is an imprint of the Taylor & Francis Group, an informa business

British Library Cataloguing-in-Publication Data
A catalogue record for this book is available from the British Library

Library of Congress Cataloging-in-Publication Data
A catalog record for this book has been requested

ISBN: 978-1-032-15638-5 (hbk)
ISBN: 978-1-032-26995-5 (pbk)
ISBN: 978-1-003-29087-2 (ebk)

DOI: 10.4324/9781003290872

Typeset in Bembo
by Apex CoVantage, LLC

Contents

1 Introduction

In early 2020, several cases of pneumonia of unknown origin were detected in Wuhan, China. Days later, its cause became known: a new coronavirus (WHO, 2020b). Weeks later, it spread to other continents, and on March 11, 2020, Tedros Adhanom, the WHO Director General, stated in a press conference that COVID-19 was considered a pandemic (WHO, 2020e). This triggered an unprecedented crisis. There were no protocols for action, and responses to previous crises were insufficient to address all of the effects of the pandemic (Ratten, 2020).

One of the main measures to stop the spread of the novel coronavirus is home confinement, meaning that one can only leave one's home to perform essential tasks such as buying basic necessities. Most educational institutions and centers were closed. Services began to be provided virtually, and teleworking became the norm. These measures forced an acceleration of the digital transformation of all sectors (Fletcher & Griffiths, 2020).

In this context, several projects have emerged that make public calls to the crowd to participate in and help address the effects of the pandemic. Their purposes are diverse ranging from raising funds to conducting scientific research on the virus. This phenomenon is called crowdsourcing and has been very useful during this period. These are projects that take place through digital platforms in which the crowd is asked to participate on a voluntary basis (Ghezzi et al., 2018).

Crowdsourcing is based on collective intelligence and has been extensively studied in the academic literature in recent years. Its fields of application include marketing, citizen science, and health, among others (Blair et al., 2019; Younis et al., 2019; Wang & Yu, 2019). It can also be used as a resource in crisis management (Yaseen & Al Omoush, 2020). Some of the advantages of this type of activity are its ability to reach large numbers of people and a reduction in the time and cost associated with a task compared to traditional methods (Paik et al., 2020; Wazny, 2018).

DOI: 10.4324/9781003290872-1

Therefore, during the initial moments of the pandemic, when solutions were urgently needed, this tool represented an alternative mean of achieving them. However, this major global crisis represented a considerable challenge. The conditions surrounding crowdsourcing were exceptional. Some were conducive to its development, and others, on the contrary, made it difficult. This may be the key to the successes and failures of certain crowdsourcing calls.

We continue to study what factors facilitate and hinder these processes (Johnson et al., 2019, Reesink et al., 2020). For this reason, studying their effect on the projects designed during this period can improve our understanding of how they work and facilitate the design of future activities. Additionally, analyzing how crowdsourcing has been employed in this context and with what objectives and what characteristics have ensured that its main elements can act in pursuit of a common objective, allowing new applications to benefit from the lessons learned during this period.

This book has several objectives. The first is to conduct a bibliographic review on the main aspects of crowdsourcing. The second is to analyze its use during the coronavirus crisis and to describe several factors that may have helped and hindered its development during this period. Finally, this book aims to analyze in detail real projects created during the early stages of the pandemic in different areas.

The book is divided into five chapters. After this introduction, Chapter 2 is dedicated to crowdsourcing. It explains the essential elements that compose these projects and other features that define them. Chapter 3 focuses on the study of crowdsourcing during the first months of the pandemic, defining its elements. A number of factors are then discussed and argued. First, it addresses factors that have been able to facilitate the success of crowdsourcing in this context, and, second, it attempts to identify other factors that have represented barriers to it. Chapter 4 analyzes four real projects created during this period and studies how the factors mentioned have affected each of them. Finally, Chapter 5 presents the conclusions of this work.

Bibliographic references

Blair, A., Key, T. M., & Wilson, M. (2019). Crowdsourcing to manage service gaps in service networks. .*Journal of Business & Industrial Marketing*, *34*(7), 1497–1505.

Fletcher, G., & Griffiths, M. (2020). Digital transformation during a lockdown. *International Journal of Information Management*, *55*, 102185.

Ghezzi, A., Gabelloni, D., Martini, A., & Natalicchio, A. (2018). Crowdsourcing: A review and suggestions for future research. *International Journal of Management Reviews*, *20*(2), 343–363.

Johnson, J. S., Fisher, G. J., & Friend, S. B. (2019). Crowdsourcing service innovation creativity: Environmental influences and contingencies. *Journal of Marketing Theory and Practice, 27*(3), 251–268.

Paik, J. H., Scholl, M., Sergeev, R., Randazzo, S., & Lakhani, K. R. (2020). Innovation contests for high-tech procurement. *Research-Technology Management, 63*(2), 36–45.

Ratten, V. (2020). Coronavirus (covid-19) and social value co-creation. *International Journal of Sociology and Social Policy*. https://doi.org/10.1108/IJSSP-06-2020-0237

Reesink, N., Hudders, L., & De Marez, L. (2020). Revisiting co-creation: Necessary success factors for crowdsourcing ideas in a consumer business setting. *Journal of Marketing and Communication, 3*(1), 95–116.

Wang, L., Xia, E., Li, H., & Wang, W. (2019). A bibliometric analysis of crowdsourcing in the field of public health. *International Journal of Environmental Research and Public Health, 16*(20), 3825.

Wazny, K. (2018). Applications of crowdsourcing in health: An overview. *Journal of Global Health, 8*(1), 010502.

World Health Organization. (2020a, January 10). *International travel and health: WHO advice on international travel and trade in relation to the outbreak of pneumonia caused by a new Coronavirus in China.* Retrieved September 10, 2020, from https://www.who.int/ith/2020-0901_outbreak_of_Pneumonia_caused_by_a_new_coronavirus_in_C/es/

World Health Organization. (2020b, March 11). *Opening address by the director-general of WHO at the press conference on COVID-19 held on 11 March 2020.* Retrieved September 10, 2020, from https://www.who.int/es/dg/speeches/detail/who-director-general-s-opening-remarks-at-the-media-briefing-on-covid-19-11-march-2020

Yaseen, S. G., & Al Omoush, K. S. (2020). Mobile crowdsourcing technology acceptance and engagement in crisis management: The case of Syrian refugees. *International Journal of Technology and Human Interaction (IJTHI), 16*(3), 1–23.

Younis, E. M., Kanjo, E., & Chamberlain, A. (2019). Designing and evaluating mobile self-reporting techniques: Crowdsourcing for citizen science. *Personal and Ubiquitous Computing, 23*(2), 329–338.

2 Crowdsourcing

2.1 Origin

Open calls have long been made for the population to carry out a certain task through collective effort. However, projects that arose before the development of information and communications technologies (ICTs) often failed because of the inability of the organizers to attract a large number of participants, the barriers that the crowd had to face to collaborate, and inertia (Kietzmann, 2017). ICTs have since allowed more people to be reached by reducing the resources needed to do so, increasing their effectiveness (Paik et al., 2020).

The concept of crowdsourcing was first described by Howe (2006a) in *Wired* magazine through different examples that illustrated the phenomenon. Months later, after extending its use, Howe (2006b) published on his personal blog the first definition of the term: "Crowdsourcing is the act of taking a job traditionally performed by a designated agent (usually an employee) and outsourcing it to an undefined, generally large group of people in the form of an open call."

Years later, academic research on the subject began, and numerous authors presented their vision of the subject, proposing their own. Estellés-Arolas and González-Ladrón-De-Guevara (2012) attempt to combine all of them and create the following integrative definition:

> Crowdsourcing is a type of participative online activity in which an individual, an institution, a non-profit organization, or company proposes to a group of individuals with varying knowledge, heterogeneity, and number, via a flexible open call, the voluntary undertaking of a task. The undertaking of the task, of variable complexity and modularity, and in which the crowd should participate bringing their work, money, knowledge and/or experience, always entails mutual benefit. The user will receive the satisfaction of a given type need,

DOI: 10.4324/9781003290872-2

be it economic, social recognition, self-esteem, or the development of individual skills, while the crowdsourcer will obtain and utilize to their advantage what the user has brought to the venture, whose form nature will depend on the type of activity undertaken.

(Estellés-Arolas & González-Ladrón-De-Guevara, 2012, p. 197)

This and other definitions that have emerged from the aggregation of common elements from various authors are too extensive. By attempting to contain as many traits as possible in one element, they do not precisely delimit what crowdsourcing is. Moreover, some academics have proposed more than one definition, increasing the confusion about the topic. Bhatti et al. (2020), criticizing these issues and trying to solve them, propose the following: "Crowdsourcing is an online distributed problem-solving paradigm, in which an individual, company, or organization publishes defined task(s) to the dynamic crowd through a flexible open call to leverage human intelligence, knowledge, skill, work and experience" (p. 4).

Song et al. (2020) highlight four characteristics of crowdsourcing: openness, dynamics, autonomy, and extensiveness. The first of these refers to the fact that people can participate through open media. The second refers to the changing character of the crowd. Autonomy represents the independence needed to actually participate. Finally, the extensiveness is related to a crowdsourcing effort's geographical dispersion. In addition, for crowdsourcing to be effective, it must be sufficiently widespread and involve the crowd (Allon & Babich, 2020). Below are the main features of its four essential elements, which are the crowdsourcer, the platform, the tasks, and the participants, and other aspects related to these projects.

2.2 Elements

2.2.1 Crowdsourcer

The crowdsourcer or requester is the agent who decides to organize a crowdsourcing activity. This allows him/her to access the talent, knowledge, information, resources, skills, and experience of the crowd, obtaining them through a single contribution or the aggregation of many of them (Guth & Brabham, 2017; Lenart-Gansiniec, 2017). It can be a public institution, company, nonprofit organization, or individual. For the former, these projects complement their activity and transform it (Torfing et al., 2019). They represent a new way of carrying out their functions and including the population in decision-making. They are used to ascertain citizens' opinions on new policies or regulations and to solicit their collaboration in carrying out public tasks, among other objectives (Apostolopoulos et al., 2018).

Lenart-Gansiniec and Sulkowski (2018) study the implementation of crowdsourcing in municipal offices. According to their research, these activities improve the quality of public services and increase the use of technology in the offices themselves to address other issues. This is an example of how this tool complements and facilitates their progress. Moreover, crowdsourcing also represents a tool that can be used by the government to build its legitimacy, empower citizens, and improve the effectiveness of public goods and services (Liu, 2017).

Crowdsourcing can be used by all companies, regardless of their size. Both large companies and small- and medium-sized enterprises can access the knowledge and resources of the crowd through these projects (Devece et al., 2019). The motivation of the crowdsourcer to lead this activity also changes over time. According to Alam and Campbell (2016), organizations that are in an exploratory stage of crowdsourcing, which have just created a call or have made a small-scale one, are usually motivated by a shortage of resources.

On the other hand, those who are in a mature stage and have experience in crowdsourcing usually do so because of their ability to achieve social commitment. These authors highlight that crowdsourcers' motivation evolves from selfishness, when they opt for crowdsourcing to be able to carry out a task thanks to the contributions of the participants at a low cost, to collectivism, representing crowdsourcing as a tool to access the experience and knowledge of the users thanks to their collaboration.

Nonprofit organizations can also benefit from crowdsourcing. It facilitates the collection of information when a disaster occurs, allowing these organizations to act more quickly and effectively (Loynes et al., 2020). It can also be used to attract new members and to reach collaborators who perform the same tasks as the volunteers of the entity in question but in a virtual way (De Wille et al., 2019). Another option is fundraising. This type of crowdsourcing is called crowdfunding. It makes it possible to collect large amounts of money by aggregating small donations. It can also be applied to carry out solidarity campaigns (Langley et al., 2020).

A crowdfunding campaign can be created by any entity, although it is especially useful for nonprofit organizations, entrepreneurs, and individuals who need funds for a cause. The search for funding is more complicated for these agents than for large companies. This can be solved thanks to the digital crowdfunding platforms that act as a loudspeaker and generate visibility for their proposals (Lacan & Desmet, 2017).

On the other hand, the crowdsourcer is responsible for drafting the call. The brief usually includes the following eight elements (Niu et al., 2019):

(1) Description of the task and the objectives pursued through it.
(2) Schedule of deadlines.
(3) Requirements that must be met by the contributions. For example, language, size, or color requirements, among others. Sometimes, a sample is attached to facilitate the understanding of these standards by future participants.
(4) Jury and awards.
(5) Criteria for choosing the winning proposal and reasons for disqualification.
(6) Requirements to be met by the crowd to participate.
(7) Other regulations that facilitate the development of ideas.
(8) Information about the crowdsourcer.

These eight elements do not have to be included in the descriptions of all calls. As an example, there are calls for which the solution is obtained by simply aggregating the contributions. In these cases, it is not necessary to decide which contribution or contributions are the winners and receive the award. Therefore, points 4 and 5 do not appear in the bases of this type of project. Another assumption is that participation is open to the entire population. Since no restrictions are established, point 6, which refers to the requirements for participation, is not included in the terms. The crowdsourcer must write the brief carefully, as it affects the development of the activity. For example, it influences the number of participants (Jiang et al., 2020), the effort they make (Yango, 2019), and the volume of quality contributions obtained (Hu et al., 2020a). Additionally, the crowdsourcer should clearly state the terms of the call to reduce the uncertainty of the crowd and attract them (Pollok et al., 2019).

On the other hand, the organizer obtains various benefits from crowdsourcing. First, through these activities, he gathers knowledge and resources from the crowd. This is the most obvious benefit, as it represents the essence of crowdsourcing. It is achieved through the contributions sent by the participants. On the other hand, crowdsourcing creates or strengthens the relationship with the individuals who respond to the call. These activities can improve the image of an entity and bring its closer to its audience. Finally, if the call focuses on the search for innovation, this process is externalized instead of being carried out internally, as has been traditionally done (Ghezzi et al., 2018).

It should also be noted that there are some barriers to the creation of a project for certain crowdsourcers. On the one hand, the entity must have sufficient digital skills to be able to do it (Gooch et al., 2020). The fact that these activities take place in a virtual environment requires that the crowdsourcers have the capacity to understand and operate in this environment. Other features that may hinder these activities are a lack of experience and the difficulty in adapting the task to be performed digitally (Thuan et al., 2016).

2.2.2 Platform

The platform is where the crowdsourcing activity takes place. It is a website or a mobile application where participants run the activity and submit their contributions. Schenk et al. (2019) identify two types of platforms: proprietary and open. Proprietary platforms are owned by the crowdsourcer, who invests resources in their creation. In addition, he or she has freedom of decision about its design, being able to adapt it to the requirements of the call. Open platforms, on the contrary, belong to a third agent. Any entity can launch a project through them. In general, the person in charge of the platform requests remuneration in exchange. They are a good alternative in various situations. For example, when an entity wants to use crowdsourcing on a one-off basis, it does not have experience in the field or does not have a community of followers (Schenk et al., 2019).

These platforms managed by a third-party agent represent a new business model. They require the payment of a fee by the crowdsourcers to place their call on the platform (Wen & Lin, 2016). Some of the factors that affect their impact include their technological infrastructure, their capacity to promote interaction between users and generate new knowledge, and their ability to motivate participation (Yuan & Hsieh, 2018). This last factor is key for these platforms. Since they obtain their benefits from the payments of the crowdsourcers, they must ensure that their calls are seen by a regular crowd of a sufficient size to be attractive.

Therefore, open platforms must design mechanisms to achieve the engagement of a community of users. If the number of members decreases, the chances of obtaining quality contributions for future calls also decrease (Schäfer et al., 2017). In such a case, the platform is less attractive for future calls since it offers access to fewer participants.

These platforms help the crowdsourcer throughout the process. For example, they offer support in formulating the problem, process the contributions before they are submitted to the organizers, and facilitate their evaluation (Diener et al., 2020). This is very useful for crowdsourcers with no previous experience. Mistakes in the planning phase can cause confusion among the crowd. Failure to adequately identify the problem and clearly and accurately state what is being requested from the crowd discourages potential participants from understanding the terms of the project (Ye & Kankanhalli, 2017).

However, a crowdsourcing activity can also take place through another alternative: social networks (Kietzmann, 2017). These platforms are often used to publicize a call and improve its scope (Ilmi et al., 2020). They can also act as the place where the call takes place. For example, Mhedhbi et al. (2019) use Facebook to collect information for scientific study. To do so, they design a questionnaire that users can answer voluntarily. These authors claim that they used this social network because it is very popular in the territory from which they want to obtain the sample.

Some social networks have functionalities that can be exploited. As an example, Hendal (2019) uses Twitter tags in a crowdsourcing project. On the other hand, these sites offer the advantage of making it easier for a large number of individuals to know about the call, since they have a large community of users. Not only are they useful for calls targeting the general population, but they are also capable of reaching very specific groups of individuals (Koo et al., 2019). In addition, they reduce the cost associated with the activity since they are free. Therefore, they represent a good alternative for entities with limited resources (Murillo-Zamorano et al., 2020).

2.2.3 Task

The task represents the work that the crowdsourcer proposes to the crowd in a project and can be of diverse nature. Komninos (2019) identifies three categories. The first is the provision of data. The participants send information that the crowdsourcer could not collect through any other method. The second consists of processing. The crowd performs small, simple tasks, such as sorting or identifying. Finally, Komninos (2019) notes that the organizer can request the generation of ideas and innovative solutions. Neto and Santos (2018) add a fourth type of task: evaluation. In this case, the result of the project consists of the resources provided by the crowdsourcer plus the evaluations of the same prepared by the crowd.

The features of the task depend on the purpose of the call itself (Rowledge, 2019). Its most studied characteristic is its complexity (Pee et al., 2018). Two main groups can be distinguished on the basis of task complexity: macrotasks and microtasks. Macrotasks represent tasks that involve a high level of difficulty and can sometimes be divided into microtasks (Kim & Robert, 2019). They are usually carried out by a crowd that is diverse in its skills. These include communication skills, creativity, and problem-solving. In addition, specialization and digital skills are sought (Lykourentzou et al., 2019). They are required in projects such as creative contests and those that request solutions to technical problems.

Microtasks, on the other hand, are tasks that are complicated to perform through computer tools but in which individuals only have to invest a few seconds or minutes to complete (Niu et al., 2019). They can consist of answering questions with yes or no options or classifying images, among others (Suzuki et al., 2019). One of the most popular microtasking platforms is Amazon Mechanical Turk (MTurk).[1] It works as a marketplace in which many people offer the option to perform simple tasks, and a large number of users access and decide which ones they want to do. Such tasks can consist of data validation, surveys, or content moderation, among others. In exchange, participants receive a small remuneration. This type of crowdsourcing is called crowdwork (Howcroft & Bergvall-Kåreborn, 2019).

Microtasks are usually combined to obtain the solution sought by the crowdsourcer (Moayedikia et al., 2020). This process is known as contribution aggregation and can be performed by him or by the platform (Tong et al., 2020). If this is to be done, it is recommended that one devise how the contributions will be combined from the first design stage (Thuan et al., 2017). In other projects, they are not aggregated since only one contribution represents the solution to the task at hand. The organizers are usually responsible for choosing which is the case for a given task. It is advisable to plan and design in advance the process that will follow this decision-making. This avoids delaying the process and, as a consequence, increasing the costs of the activity (Christensen & Karlsson, 2019).

It should be noted that some problems may arise in this context. For example, participants are disadvantaged by asymmetric information since they do not know the preferences of the crowdsourcer. This acts against the optimal functioning of the process. In view of this, the crowdsourcer can comment on the participants' contributions. Such an approach reduces their uncertainty and increases their effort in developing proposals (Jiang and Wang, 2020).

Another option is to design a new crowdsourcing activity to delegate the election of the winner to the crowd (Neto & Santos, 2018). This practice helps to attract a greater volume of participants in innovation competitions (Chen et al., 2020). In addition, it can be used to give recognition to the most experienced users of the platform and thus prevent them from leaving it. To this end, greater weight can be applied to the assessments of these participants (Chen et al., 2020b).

Sometimes the task must be carried out in a specific location, or the location is part of the value of the contribution itself. This is called spatial crowdsourcing. It is often participated in through mobile devices because it requires moving through the physical world. Therefore, it generates more concern than other types of activities with respect to maintaining user privacy (Liu et al., 2018). Most of these projects call for microtasking, although others increase the level of difficulty of the work (Gao et al., 2017).

2.2.4 Participants

The participants are that part of the population that decides to contribute in a project. These individuals are self-selected (Flostrand, 2017). In other words, they intervene voluntarily. The crowdsourcer launches a call, and those interested respond to it. Therefore, it is not known in advance how many users will participate (à Campo et al., 2019). This makes them a heterogeneous group of people with different levels of knowledge and experience (Moayedikia et al., 2019). To participate, the crowd must have resources such as time and technical infrastructure (e.g., a device to access the platform and Internet connection), the ability to perform the task properly, and the motivation to do so (Bal et al., 2017; Wehn & Almomani, 2019).

Additionally, sometimes participants must possess certain skills to be able to execute a task properly. This usually goes hand in hand with the level of complexity of the work. Macrotasks require the participation of individuals with specific skills. Microtasks, on the other hand, can be executed by a nonspecialist crowd (Lykourentzou et al., 2019). Thus, the crowd may refer to the general population or a group within it.

Sometimes, potential participants are asked to demonstrate possession of such skills. To do so, they require some kind of certificate or take a pretest. In others, on the contrary, no screening is done, even if the task involves a high degree of difficulty. In other words, certain skills are needed to perform the task, but they do not have to be demonstrated beforehand. In these cases, the subsequent quality control takes on particular importance. The contributions must be subjected to an examination to verify that they meet the established technical requirements. This strategy, although it may increase the cost because it increases the time and resources devoted to the project, can be useful. High-quality contributions come from both highly skilled and less-skilled participants (Hu et al., 2020a). There is also another alternative for the crowdsourcer.

It consists of designing a training that future participants must complete before collaborating if they lack the required skills (Komninos, 2019). Both measures increase the number of participants in the call, since it is less restrictive. In this way, a larger number of contributions are obtained.

However, these restrictions are not exclusive to projects that require specific skills. Other calls may also be established on the basis of other characteristics, such as experience, location, or professional activity (Frewin & Church, 2019; Urra & Ilarri, 2019). In these cases, selective calls are made, allowing only a few individuals from the crowd to participate (de Mattos et al., 2018). Although fewer contributions are made, their quality can be higher (Acar, 2019). Therefore, the crowd-sourcer must weigh whether it will be more beneficial to open or restrict access. One category within the selective call that has been investigated in academic research is internal crowdsourcing. Such efforts are called by a particular company, and the crowd they address consists of its employees. It should be noted that the project may be open to all employees or restricted to certain groups such as a department (Pohlisch, 2020).

On the other hand, participation can be done individually or collectively. On the basis of the interdependence between users, Renard and Davis (2019) distinguish three forms of participation. The first is competition. In this case, the crowd competes for a limited number of rewards. Participants' performance is subject to a set of rules during the process, and the interactions between them are controlled. Moreover, in its strictest form, there is no contact between users (Sari et al., 2019). Contests are examples of competitive crowdsourcing. The second modality is cooperation. It is characterized by connection between participants. Several of them share a common goal. They are governed by implicit rules, distributing resources among users. The communication between them flows openly. This last point is crucial to facilitate collaboration between several participants. Therefore, it is advisable to include on the platform a tool that allows both communication between two users and between all members of a team (Niu et al., 2019). Finally, there is co-opetition, which arises from the combination of the two previous approaches. In these projects, interdependence between users at the individual level is encouraged. Participants need community support to achieve their goals. The aim is to create a climate of exchange, although participants compete with each other. This is because to win, they must obtain a positive evaluation from others (Renard & Davis, 2019).

Participants can play different roles in crowdsourcing, from being problem-solvers to community members (Troll et al., 2019). Different authors have proposed classifications of participants using different factors to make this division and differentiating the category of crowdsourcing to which they refer. For example, Fuger et al. (2017) identify five roles that users of crowdsourcing virtual communities can play based on the volume of comments and contributions they make. Gadiraju and Zhuang (2019) propose a classification of macrotask crowdsourcing participants based on their type of motivation, the time they take to complete the task and their accuracy.

Finally, participants can collaborate actively by preparing contributions or, conversely, passively. In the latter case, the contributions are collected through the sensors embedded in the mobile devices of the crowd. Huang et al. (2017) call them participatory and opportunistic contribution. And projects that request opportunistic contributions are called crowdsensing. In this category of crowdsourcing, individuals play a passive role, and the task is carried out through the sensors in their mobile devices. Its main application is environmental monitoring (Vianna et al., 2020). In this case, the tasks are spatial-temporal. That is, they are linked to the location of the subject and the time at which the information is sent (Wang et al., 2018).

2.3 Other aspects

2.3.1 Scope and duration

After creating a project, the crowdsourcer must make it known to attract participants. This can be done through his or her own means or delegated to another agent. Specifically, when using an open platform, the user community that this intermediary has is accessed. Although it facilitates outreach, participation may not take place if these individuals do not have any link to the crowdsourcer or the incentives are not motivating (Dahlander et al., 2019). In this case, as in the case of proprietary platforms, the crowdsourcer can carry out its own communication actions. An adequate communication strategy is key to the success of a call (Van Galen, 2019). For this purpose, it is possible to use social networks and disseminate through informal networks or direct invitations (Ilmi et al., 2020).

The scope of a crowdsourcing project also depends on other factors. For example, the number of individuals who can participate in selective calls is smaller than in the case of activities without participation restrictions. Additionally, a platform may not be accessible from a particular country. This is common in the case of mobile applications. Another barrier to reach is language. A project can allow the collaboration of any individual, but if he or she does not know the language in which it is written, it is impossible for him or her to send a contribution. Another case is that of spatial crowdsourcing. Since it depends on the user's location, the chances of a person participating are also lower.

On the other hand, a project may have a defined duration or be designed to be long term. In other words, it can have a deadline by which it comes to an end or it can remain active for an indefinite period. An example of crowdsourcing with an end date is contests. In these, the organizer sets a period for sending contributions. When this period ends, the proposals are evaluated, and the winner is chosen (Segev, 2020). It is necessary to establish a deadline to stop receiving proposals. One particular case is hackathons. These are events of short duration, generally few days, in which individuals from different disciplines and with different experiences collaborate toward a common end (Pulay & Asino, 2019). Although these activities are traditionally carried out in a face-to-face fashion, they can also be referred to as short-term crowdsourcing projects (Tang et al., 2018; Tucker et al., 2018).

When no deadline is set, the project is intended to remain active and receive contributions over the long term. Sometimes, it becomes a virtual community (Kohler & Chesbrough, 2019). In these communities, participants collaborate on an ongoing basis and often interact with each other. They resemble a social network (Fuger et al., 2017). In addition, the figure of the moderator emerges. These are agents who monitor the activity within the platform to ensure its proper functioning. This work can be done by the participants when they achieve a certain status (à Campo et al., 2019). These projects require the participation of the crowd to continue to exist. Therefore, effective incentive mechanisms must be designed to ensure that contributions are made on a long-term basis.

In both cases, regardless of whether a deadline is set, a maximum number of contributions per participant can be set. However, it is more common for this restriction to exist in calls of defined duration. Soliman and Tuunainen (2015) distinguish between recurring and nonrecurring tasks. The latter are unique. That is, the crowdsourcer only requires one contribution from each participant. Recurrent tasks, on the other hand, occur when the crowdsourcer asks for help from the crowd to perform tasks on a regular basis.

Wang and Yu (2020) define sustainable crowdsourcing as the approach followed by crowdsourcers who frequently employ crowdsourcing as a strategy within their innovation activities. It is based on continuous interactions over time between crowdsourcer and crowd, rather than creating a one-off call to solve a particular technical problem. The platform must be adapted to this and have an appropriate design and technical support that allows a participant to send more than one contribution if the tasks are recurring.

On the other hand, creating recurring tasks can be beneficial to the crowdsourcer. According to Dissanayake et al. (2018), participants act strategically and make the greatest effort when the call is nearing its end. Therefore, they recommend dividing the project into shorter phases to increase user performance throughout the process. This occurs when participants can send more than one contribution. In fact, participants who enter the process late devote less effort to it than those who enter it early, especially if a large incentive is offered in return (Deodhar, 2020). Therefore, dividing a task into smaller tasks to be performed successively in exchange for small remuneration may result in greater effort on the part of the participants. In this way, the quality of the activity is increased.

These platforms also face a challenge: how to keep users actively engaged over time (Komninos, 2019). The following positively affect the intention to continue participating: perceived fairness (Liu & Liu, 2019; Wang et al., 2019), interaction with other users (Wang et al., 2019), incentives such as reputation systems (Xiao & Ke, 2019), motivation and perceived control of behavior (Liang et al., 2017), and communication (Schäfer et al., 2017).

Finally, it should be noted that in the case of platforms that host successive competitions from the same crowdsourcer, problems may arise. If a user's contribution is not selected as the winner of a contest, it may discourage the development of proposals for future calls. According to Piezunka and Dahlander (2019), this can be avoided through communication. In particular, explicit notifications and explanations for why a user has not been chosen influences his or her intention to participate again in a positive way.

2.3.2 Incentive

The organizers of a crowdsourcing project should encourage the crowd to enter it. They can do this before participation (e.g., by sending an invitation email), during participation (e.g., by facilitating communication), and after the deadline for sending contributions. The last encouragement they can provide is rewards for having done the work (Troll et al., 2019).

Monetary rewards represent the most common type of incentive in these activities (Bakici, 2020). They can encourage participation regardless of whether the task is complex (Si et al., 2020) or simple (Phuttharak & Loke, 2020). However, the amount should be established with caution. According to Acar (2018), sufficiently high monetary rewards attract more participants in creative crowdsourcing. However, they bring in the same number of ideas regardless of whether there is a monetary reward. In addition, ideas are more original and novel if no monetary reward is offered, but they are more useful if the reward is high. In other words, high-value financial rewards attract more participants whose contributions are more appropriate. However, if the crowdsourcer wants to collect a large number of contributions from each participant, the best strategy is not to establish a monetary incentive.

In any case, Acar (2018) shows that the amount should never be less than the sum the crowd considers appropriate since it is less effective than either of the other two alternatives and entails a loss of resources. The problem in applying these results in a practical way lies in how to determine what amount is adequate for the crowd. This depends on factors such as the level of competence, the task to be performed or the need for specific skills to carry it out (Acar, 2018). On the other hand, offering just one or a few prizes is a common practice when crowdsourcing takes place in the form of a contest. Although its aim is to encourage participation, it can have the opposite effect. Members of the crowd may make little effort in developing their contribution or even decide not to participate if they believe that the chance of winning is too low. Although the level of effort can also be low if many rewards are established, participants may believe that even some poor-quality contributions will be rewarded (Ales et al., 2017).

There are other types of incentives beyond monetary rewards that are also effective. Some of them appeal to the personal growth of the individual. This is the case when activities offer the possibility of developing skills or contributing new knowledge. They represent a way to use leisure time for productive work (Deng & Koshi, 2016). Another alternative is to link the project to the realization of a good for the community. According to Cappa et al. (2019), the possibility of contributing to a social cause has a positive influence on participation. These authors argue that contributing a benefit to society can increase self-esteem and satisfaction, motivating the collaboration of the crowd.

Mechanisms can also be created to provide entertainment for users (Brovelli et al., 2018). However, it is not always necessary to create specific mechanisms to make the activity seem fun to them. Despite the limited attention given to it, performing the task itself can make users enjoy themselves and attract participation (Ahmad et al., 2017). Reputation systems can also be very useful for calls that are intended to last over the long term. Individuals often remain engaged when they feel that their work matters and that they are valued within the community (Van Galen, 2019).

The type of incentive used depends on the problem and the traits of the participants (Allahbakhsh et al., 2019). In the planning phase, before the activity takes place, it is necessary to identify which segment of the public one wants to attract and what their needs are (Van Galen, 2019). In this way, the appropriate incentive mechanism can be implemented. Even so, it should be noted that this is somewhat complicated given the complexity involved in analyzing user motivation (Liang et al., 2018).

The appropriate incentives also depend on the duration of the project. Achieving the engagement of the crowd in the long term is a challenge for crowdsourcers (Soon & Saguy, 2017). Their motivation has to be analyzed in both the short and long terms, as it can vary (Morschheuser & Hamari, 2019). The effect of some incentives has been studied specifically in long-term activities. Providing feedback and highlighting the impact of contributions make it easier for participants who contribute altruistically to continue to show interest in the activity (Baruch et al., 2016).

When a call is created that is intended to become a community where knowledge is exchanged in the long term, voting and commentary systems for users take on special importance. According to Chen et al. (2019), obtaining positive votes and comments from other members encourages continued contribution. Participants feel valued by the community, as well as a sense of responsibility toward it and toward continuing to share knowledge. Negative votes, on the other hand, demotivate users and encourage their abandonment. However, these mechanisms are not appropriate for all projects intended to last over the long term. In contests and challenges where participants compete for a reward instead of a space to share knowledge, user voting can be counterproductive. On the one hand, they may value other members negatively out of envy for their success. On the other hand, members may support those with whom they have ties of friendship, even if their proposal is not a quality one (Faullant & Dolfus, 2017). These communities benefit from social support among their members. According to Ihl et al. (2020), voting makes users feel identified with the group and gives meaning to the experience, which facilitates their engagement to the project.

Finally, it should be noted that a user ceasing to participate after performing one or more tasks is not the only concern in this context. A fairly widespread and little-studied problem is the abandonment of the activity when the contribution has been started but not yet completed (Han et al., 2019). In these cases, the participant's effort is not visible to the crowdsourcer since he or she gives up before sending his or her proposal and there is no possibility that the work will be rewarded. In other words, the resources invested in the intervention are wasted.

2.3.3 Ethics and privacy

There are some circumstances regarding the ethics of crowdsourcing that generate controversy. These are usually related to financial rewards. On the one hand, projects that offer monetary rewards to one or a few participants are under discussion. Only those who, according to the organizer, have sent the best or most appropriate contributions are rewarded. Some question whether it is ethical to not reward the rest of the participants (Liu & Shestak, 2020). Winning depends as much on one's performance as it does on the competitors (Mo et al., 2018). In addition, participants may feel undervalued and thus not contribute (Sheehan & Pittman, 2019).

Wang and Yu (2019) recommend that participants in this type of call pay attention to other elements they offer, such as the possibility of acquiring knowledge and experience or developing new skills. These authors argue that these elements improve the competitiveness of users, which will allow them to win future calls. Moreover, according to Zhang et al. (2019), participants with less learning ability tend to prefer high monetary rewards and win, on average, fewer crowdsourcing contests. In contrast, those with greater ability value them less. The former may attempt to avoid contributing to contests involving highly skilled competitors. However, Zhang et al. (2019) recommend confronting them since this serves as a lesson and leads to an improvement in their skills. In this way, the skills needed to win competitions in the long term are acquired.

On the other hand, some authors understand crowdwork, in which simple tasks are performed in exchange for a small remuneration, as a job in itself. They argue that participants in these platforms should not be seen as individuals who voluntarily perform a task for altruism or entertainment but should be treated as employees and remunerated accordingly (Martin et al., 2017). This may even be seen as a form of modern exploitation for which no specific legal regulation exists (Schlagwein et al., 2019)

Other authors defend this type of crowdsourcing. According to Fieseler et al. (2019), most crowdsourcing participants positively value the opportunity that these activities offer to earn additional income. Regarding the criticism about the destruction of jobs through such outsourcing, Fieseler et al. (2019) argue that these projects create new jobs. And Apostolopoulos et al. (2018) argue that these collaborative activities should be seen as a support rather than a threat by professionals.

Another problem lies in the management of the intellectual property rights of the contributions. This affects both those relating to the winning contributions, if it is a competition, and those of all the others (Dahlander et al., 2019). The crowdsourcer establishes whether all the rights or only those of the selected proposals are transferred to him or her. This is an abusive practice since it gives organizers the right to use the ideas of participants who have not received a reward for their effort. However, if the rules are too lax, it may be difficult for the organizer to benefit from the ideas submitted by users. If they are too strict, this may discourage participation (Tekic & Willoughby, 2020). The management of such rules has been widely studied in the academic literature, but there is no consensus or model to follow (Liu & Shestak, 2020).

The organizers of these activities also have to display fair behavior. This becomes especially important when crowdsourcing is applied to policy making within the new trend toward open government. It represents a strategy to involve citizens in decision-making, pursuing inclusion, and equality for all individuals. However, this may not be the case in practice. According to Chen and Aitamurto (2019), all contributions are not equally valued, and some are more likely to receive a response. This can be the case when the volume of proposals received is very high. If the government does not have the resources to analyze and evaluate all of them, some are left unattended. Those that attract the most attention are those that have support from groups that collaborate with public authorities and those that are perceived as more viable. All of this undermines the democratic nature of these calls (Chen & Aitamurto, 2019).

The crowdsourcer must also ensure that the crowd will not be harmed as a result of participation. To this end, he or she must establish a security policy that guarantees participants' protection (Hosseini et al., 2015). Crowdsourcing platforms can be vulnerable to cyberattacks, particularly platforms that host personal information of participants, such as their gender and age (Hassan & Rahim, 2017). Xia & McKernan (2020) argue that to ensure that privacy is preserved in crowdsourcing, the measures taken by the crowdsourcer must be controlled.

They recommend the encryption of sensitive data provided by the participants and the inspection of the security and responsibilities of the agent who launches the call. In addition, they emphasize the importance of transparency. The crowdsourcer must inform about the future use of the information provided by the users and allow its withdrawal if a participant requires it. It should be noted that despite the efforts of the organizers to protect participants, privacy and cybersecurity must continue to be enhanced for all types of collaborative activities taking place over the Internet (Papangelis et al., 2019).

2.3.4 Control mechanisms

Crowdsourcing quality is affected by various factors, such as the crowd-sourcer, the participants, the platform, the task, the complexity of the problem, the incentive system, and the evaluation of the contributions (Hu et al., 2020b; Shergadwala et al., 2020). Additionally, the crowd participating is heterogeneous, with dispersed locations and different levels of experience, which can lead to problems (Niu et al., 2018). Some of the reasons that participants submit low-quality contributions are a lack of experience, a failure to understand the requirements of the call, or dishonest behavior to achieve a benefit (Allahbakhsh et al., 2019). Therefore, the crowdsourcer should monitor the whole process, evaluating the contributions received or answering the questions of the participants (Lenart-Gansiniec, 2017). However, sometimes, the platform is responsible for such functions, especially in the case of open platforms, which can offer control functions.

Pinto et al. (2019) divide the control mechanisms used in crowdsourcing to ensure the quality of contributions into four categories: pessimistic, optimistic, feedback-based, and incentive-based. In the case of pessimistic mechanisms, quality is assured through direct identification of fraudulent participants. When the system detects that a user is behaving in a misleading way, it excludes him/her. No distinction is usually made between users, and they are all subject to the same controls (Pinto et al., 2019). These include various methods for measuring user behavior and estimating the quality of their contributions, such as the time they spend on the platform or the number of times they click. However, they are not very useful as control mechanisms when the task to be performed is very simple, since the volume of behavior that can be derived and analyzed from such tasks is very low. Therefore, the accuracy of the predictions is low (Suzuki et al., 2019).

One of the most popular pessimistic mechanisms is the golden question (Checco et al., 2020). It is widely used in crowdwork. Since micro-tasking is rewarded with a small fee, participants may engage in malicious behavior to gain more profit. These are questions for which the answers have been previously established. The crowdworker does not know this information and answers the question as if it were the crowdsourcing task. The response is compared to the preestablished response. In this way, the rigor and precision of participants' work can be contrasted. Answering the question is not part of the work entrusted by the crowd-sourcer but rather represents a mechanism for controlling participation. This improves the validity and reliability of the contributions (Cabrall et al., 2018).

Optimistic mechanisms ensure the adequacy of contributions by aggregating them. Unlike the above, such mechanisms usually recognize that two participants may have different skills or capabilities. Therefore, they attempt to recognize the best and assign different weights to their contributions in the aggregation process (Pinto et al., 2019). In the literature, there are various proposals regarding the application of algorithms to estimate the quality and experience of the participants. However, they present some limitations, such as the increase in the cost of the activity or its basis on erroneous assumptions, such as that each individual will solve all the tasks proposed to him or her (Moayedikia et al., 2019). Other options include taking a pluralistic approach and giving equal weight to all and weighing the opinions of participants based on their ability or self-confidence (Saab et al., 2019).

Feedback methods are based on monitoring the actions of the participants within the platform and communication. As with optimistic mechanisms, they recognize those who perform best (Pinto et al., 2019). Previous results are analyzed to predict future behavior. However, to do this, the activity must be of adequate duration. If it is too short, the data on which the analysis is based may be insufficient. Additionally, in these calls, it is important to bear in mind that a participant's performance may vary over time. Therefore, Shi et al. (2019) recommend introducing mechanisms to assess performance dynamically.

Finally, those based on incentives guarantee the quality of contributions through motivation (Pinto et al., 2019). There is no research on this subject, but its usefulness could be limited. For example, participants may engage in malicious behavior to obtain greater rewards. If there is no other control mechanism and rewards are only given for performing the task without verifying its validity, users may send useless proposals that do not meet the minimum quality requirements. They can also contribute in duplicate to enrich themselves (Chen et al., 2018). Moreover, some members of the crowd participate with dishonest motivations to harm the call itself, mocking it (Wilson et al., 2017).

Note

1   www.mturk.com

Bibliographic references

À Campo, S., Khan, V. J., Papangelis, K., & Markopoulos, P. (2019). Community heuristics for user interface evaluation of crowdsourcing platforms. *Future Generation Computer Systems*, *95*, 775–789.

Acar, O. A. (2018). Harnessing the creative potential of consumers: Money, participation, and creativity in idea crowdsourcing. *Marketing Letters, 29*(2), 177–188.

Acar, O. A. (2019). Motivations and solution appropriateness in crowdsourcing challenges for innovation. *Research Policy, 48*(8), 103716.

Ahmad, R., Mahmod, M., Chit, S. C., Na'in, N., Habbal, A., & Wiwied, V. (2017). More than money matters: Examining motivational factors for participating in crowdsourcing platform. *Advanced Science Letters, 23*(5), 4310–4313.

Alam, S. L., & Campbell, J. (2016). Understanding the temporality of organizational motivation for crowdsourcing. *Scandinavian Journal of Information Systems, 28*(1), 91–120.

Ales, L., Cho, S. H., & Körpeoğlu, E. (2017). Optimal award scheme in innovation tournaments. *Operations Research, 65*(3), 693–702.

Allahbakhsh, M., Arbabi, S., Galavii, M., Daniel, F., & Benatallah, B. (2019). Crowdsourcing planar facility location allocation problems. *Computing, 101*(3), 237–261.

Allon, G., & Babich, V. (2020). Crowdsourcing and crowdfunding in the manufacturing and services sectors. *Manufacturing & Service Operations Management, 22*(1), 102–112.

Apostolopoulos, K., Geli, M., Petrelli, P., Potsiou, C., & Ioannidis, C. (2018). A new model for cadastral surveying using crowdsourcing. *Survey Review, 50*(359), 122–133.

Bakici, T. (2020). Comparison of crowdsourcing platforms from social-psychological and motivational perspectives. *International Journal of Information Management, 54*, 102121.

Bal, A. S., Weidner, K., Hanna, R., & Mills, A. J. (2017). Crowdsourcing and brand control. *Business Horizons, 60*(2), 219–228.

Baruch, A., May, A., & Yu, D. (2016). The motivations, enablers and barriers for voluntary participation in an online crowdsourcing platform. *Computers in Human Behavior, 64*, 923–931.

Bhatti, S. S., Gao, X., & Chen, G. (2020). General framework, opportunities and challenges for crowdsourcing techniques: A comprehensive survey. *Journal of Systems and Software, 167*, 110611.

Brovelli, M. A., Celino, I., Fiano, A., Molinari, M. E., & Venkatachalam, V. (2018). A crowdsourcing-based game for land cover validation. *Applied Geomatics, 10*, 1–11.

Cabrall, C. D., Lu, Z., Kyriakidis, M., Manca, L., Dijksterhuis, C., Happee, R., & de Winter, J. (2018). Validity and reliability of naturalistic driving scene categorization judgments from crowdsourcing. *Accident Analysis & Prevention, 114*, 25–33.

Cappa, F., Rosso, F., & Hayes, D. (2019). Monetary and social rewards for crowdsourcing. *Sustainability, 11*(10), 2834.

Checco, A., Bates, J., & Demartini, G. (2020). Adversarial attacks on crowdsourcing quality control. *Journal of Artificial Intelligence Research, 67*, 375–408.

Chen, K., & Aitamurto, T. (2019). Barriers for crowd's impact in crowdsourced policymaking: Civic data overload and filter hierarchy. *International Public Management Journal, 22*(1), 99–126.

Chen, L., Baird, A., & Straub, D. (2019). Why do participants continue to contribute? Evaluation of usefulness voting and commenting motivational affordances within an online knowledge community. *Decision Support Systems, 118*, 21–32.

Chen, L., Xu, P., & Liu, D. (2020). Effect of crowd voting on participation in crowdsourcing contests. *Journal of Management Information Systems, 37*(2), 510–535.

Chen, P. P., Sun, H. L., Fang, Y. L., & Huai, J. P. (2018). Collusion-proof result inference in crowdsourcing. *Journal of Computer Science and Technology, 33*(2), 351–365.

Christensen, I., & Karlsson, C. (2019). Open innovation and the effects of crowdsourcing in a pharma ecosystem. *Journal of Innovation & Knowledge, 4*(4), 240–247.

Dahlander, L., Jeppesen, L. B., & Piezunka, H. (2019). How organizations manage crowds: Define, broadcast, attract, and select. *Managing Inter-Organizational Collaborations: Process Views (Research in the Sociology of Organizations, 64*, 239–270, Emerald Publishing Limited.

de Mattos, C. A., Kissimoto, K. O., & Laurindo, F. J. B. (2018). The role of information technology for building virtual environments to integrate crowdsourcing mechanisms into the open innovation process. *Technological Forecasting and Social Change, 129*, 143–153.

Deng, X. N., & Joshi, K. D. (2016). Why individuals participate in micro-task crowdsourcing work environment: Revealing crowdworkers' perceptions. *Journal of the Association for Information Systems, 17*(10), 711–736.

Deodhar, S. (2021). Different eyes on the same prize: Implications of entry timing hetero geneity and incentives for contestant effort in innovation tournament. *Information Technology & People, 34*(2), 526–556.

Devece, C., Palacios, D., & Ribeiro-Navarrete, B. (2019). The effectiveness of crowdsourcing in knowledge-based industries: The moderating role of transformational leadership and organisational learning. *Economic Research-Ekonomska istraživanja, 32*(1), 335–351.

De Wille, T., Schäler, R., Exton, C., & Exton, G. (2019). Crowdsourcing localisation for non-profit projects: The client perspective. *The Journal of Internationalization and Localization, 6*(1), 45–67.

Diener, K., Luettgens, D., & Piller, F. T. (2020). Intermediation for open innovation: Comparing direct versus delegated search strategies of innovation intermediaries. *International Journal of Innovation Management, 24*(4), 2050037.

Dissanayake, I., Zhang, J., Yasar, M., & Nerur, S. P. (2018). Strategic effort allocation in online innovation tournaments. *Information & Management, 55*(3), 396–406.

Estellés-Arolas, E., & González-Ladrón-De-Guevara, F. (2012). Towards an integrated crowdsourcing definition. *Journal of Information Science, 38*(2), 189–200.

Faullant, R., & Dolfus, G. (2017). Everything community? Destructive processes in communities of crowdsourcing competitions. *Business Process Management Journal, 23*(6), 1108–1128.

Fieseler, C., Bucher, E., & Hoffmann, C. P. (2019). Unfairness by design? The perceived fairness of digital labor on crowdworking platforms. *Journal of Business Ethics, 156*(4), 987–1005.

Flostrand, A. (2017). Finding the future: Crowdsourcing versus the Delphi technique. *Business Horizons, 60*(2), 229–236.

Frewin, S., & Church, S. (2019). Midwives' evaluation of their role in crowdsourcing activities to improve the maternity experience: Part 2. *British Journal of Midwifery, 27*(7), 420–426.

Fuger, S., Schimpf, R., Füller, J., & Hutter, K. (2017). User roles and team structures in a crowdsourcing community for international development-a social network perspective. *Information Technology for Development, 23*(3), 438–462.

Gadiraju, U., & Zhuang, M. (2019). What you sow, so shall you reap! Toward preselection mechanisms for macrotask crowdsourcing. In *Macrotask crowdsourcing: Engaging the crowds to address complex problems* (pp. 163–188). Cham: Springer.

Gao, D., Tong, Y., She, J., Song, T., Chen, L., & Xu, K. (2017). Top-k team recommendation and its variants in spatial crowdsourcing. *Data Science and Engineering, 2*(2), 136–150.

Ghezzi, A., Gabelloni, D., Martini, A., & Natalicchio, A. (2018). Crowdsourcing: A review and suggestions for future research. *International Journal of Management Reviews*, 20(2), 343–363.

Gooch, D., Kelly, R. M., Stiver, A., van der Linden, J., Petre, M., Richards, M., . . . Walton, C. (2020). The benefits and challenges of using crowdfunding to facilitate community-led projects in the context of digital civics. *International Journal of Human-Computer Studies*, 134, 33–43.

Guth, K. L., & Brabham, D. C. (2017). Finding the diamond in the rough: Exploring communication and platform in crowdsourcing performance. *Communication Monographs*, 84(4), 510–533.

Han, L., Roitero, K., Gadiraju, U., Sarasua, C., Checco, A., Maddalena, E., & Demartini, G. (2021). The impact of task abandonment in crowdsourcing. *IEEE Transactions on Knowledge and Data Engineering*, 33(5), 2266–2279.

Hassan, N. H., & Rahim, F. A. (2017). The rise of crowdsourcing using social media platforms: Security and privacy issues. *Pertanika Journal of Science & Technology*, 25, 79–88.

Hendal, B. (2019). Hashtags as crowdsourcing: A case study of Arabic hashtags on Twitter. *Social Networking*, 8(4), 158–173.

Hosseini, M., Shahri, A., Phalp, K., Taylor, J., & Ali, R. (2015). Crowdsourcing: A taxonomy and systematic mapping study. *Computer Science Review*, 17, 43–69.

Howcroft, D., & Bergvall-Kåreborn, B. (2019). A typology of crowdwork platforms. *Work, Employment and Society*, 33(1), 21–38.

Howe, J. (2006a). The rise of crowdsourcing. *Wired Magazine*. Retrieved September 27, 2020, from https://www.wired.com/2006/06/crowds

Howe, J. (2006b). *Crowdsourcing: A definition*. Retrieved September 27, 2020, from https://crowdsourcing.typepad.com/cs/2006/06/crowdsourcing_a.html

Hu, F., Bijmolt, T. H., & Huizingh, E. K. (2020a). The impact of innovation contest briefs on the quality of solvers and solutions. *Technovation*, 90–91, 102099.

Hu, Z., Wu, W., Luo, J., Wang, X., & Li, B. (2020b). Quality assessment in competition-based software crowdsourcing. *Frontiers of Computer Science*, 14(6), 1–14.

Huang, Y., Shema, A., & Xia, H. (2017). A proposed genome of mobile and situated crowdsourcing and its design implications for encouraging contributions. *International Journal of Human-Computer Studies*, 102, 69–80.

Ihl, A., Strunk, K. S., & Fiedler, M. (2020). The mediated effects of social support in professional online communities on crowdworker engagement in micro-task crowdworking. *Computers in Human Behavior*, 113, 106482.

Ilmi, Z., Wijaya, A., Kasuma, J., & Darma, D. C. (2020). The crowdsourcing data for innovation. *European Journal of Management Issues*, 28(1–2), 3–12.

Jiang, J., & Wang, Y. (2020). A theoretical and empirical investigation of feedback in ideation contests. *Production and Operations Management*, 29(2), 481–500.

Jiang, Z., Huang, Y., & Beil, D. R. (2021). The role of problem specification in crowdsourcing contests for design problems: A theoretical and empirical analysis. *Manufacturing & Service Operations Management*, 23(3), 637–656.

Kietzmann, J. H. (2017). Crowdsourcing: A revised definition and introduction to new research. *Business Horizons*, 60(2), 151–153.

Kim, S., & Robert Jr, L. P. (2019). Crowdsourcing coordination: A review and research agenda for crowdsourcing. In *Macrotask crowdsourcing: Engaging the crowds to address complex problems* (pp. 1–43). Cham: Springer.

Kohler, T., & Chesbrough, H. (2019). From collaborative community to competitive market: The quest to build a crowdsourcing platform for social innovation. *R&D Management, 49*(3), 356–368.

Komninos, A. (2019). Pro-social behaviour in crowdsourcing systems: Experiences from a field deployment for beach monitoring. *International Journal of Human-Computer Studies, 124*, 93–115.

Koo, K., Shee, K., & Gormley, E. A. (2019). Following the crowd: Patterns of crowdsourcing on Twitter among urologists. *World Journal of Urology, 37*(3), 567–572.

Lacan, C., & Desmet, P. (2017). Does the crowdfunding platform matter? Risks of negative attitudes in two-sided markets. *Journal of Consumer Marketing, 34*(6), 472–479.

Langley, P., Lewis, S., McFarlane, C., Painter, J., & Vradis, A. (2020). Crowdfunding cities: Social entrepreneurship, speculation and solidarity in Berlin. *Geoforum, 115*, 11–20.

Lenart-Gansiniec, R. (2017). Virtual knowledge sharing in crowdsourcing: Measurement dilemmas. *Journal of Entrepreneurship, Management and Innovation, 13*(3), 95–124.

Lenart-Gansiniec, R., & Sulkowski, L. (2018). Crowdsourcing-a new paradigm of organizational learning of public organizations. *Sustainability, 10*(10), 3359.

Liang, B., Huang, X., & Jiang, J. (2017). Research on antecedent factors of solvers' continuous participation in crowdsourcing logistics. *Journal of Business Economics, 37*(7), 5–15.

Liang, H., Wang, M. M., Wang, J. J., & Xue, Y. (2018). How intrinsic motivation and extrinsic incentives affect task effort in crowdsourcing contests: A mediated moderation model. *Computers in Human Behavior, 81*, 168–176.

Liu, A., Wang, W., Shang, S., Li, Q., & Zhang, X. (2018). Efficient task assignment in spatial crowdsourcing with worker and task privacy protection. *GeoInformatica, 22*(2), 335–362.

Liu, H. K. (2017). Crowdsourcing government: Lessons from multiple disciplines. *Public Administration Review, 77*(5), 656–667.

Liu, Y., & Liu, Y. (2019). The effect of workers' justice perception on continuance participation intention in the crowdsourcing market. *Internet Research, 29*(6), 1485–1508.

Liu, Z., & Shestak, V. (2020). Issues of crowdsourcing and mobile app development through the intellectual property protection of third parties. *Peer-to-Peer Networking and Applications, 14*(5).

Loynes, C., Ouenniche, J., & De Smedt, J. (2020). The detection and location estimation of disasters using Twitter and the identification of Non-Governmental Organisations using crowdsourcing. *Annals of Operations Research*, 1–33.

Lykourentzou, I., Khan, V. J., Papangelis, K., & Markopoulos, P. (2019). Macrotask crowdsourcing: An integrated definition. In *Macrotask crowdsourcing: Engaging the crowds to address complex problems* (pp. 1–13). Cham: Springer.

Martin, D., Carpendale, S., Gupta, N., Hoßfeld, T., Naderi, B., Redi, J., . . . Wechsung, I. (2017). Understanding the crowd: Ethical and practical matters in the academic use of crowdsourcing. In *Evaluation in the crowd: Crowdsourcing and human-centered experiments* (pp. 27–69). Cham: Springer.

Mhedhbi, Z., Masson, V., Hidalgo, J., & Haouès-Jouve, S. (2019). Collection of refined architectural parameters by crowdsourcing using Facebook social network: Case of Greater Tunis. *Urban Climate, 29*, 100499.

Mo, J., Sarkar, S., & Menon, S. (2018). Know when to run: Recommendations in crowdsourcing contests. *MIS Quarterly, 42*(3), 919–944.

Moayedikia, A., Yeoh, W., Ong, K. L., & Boo, Y. L. (2019). Improving accuracy and lowering cost in crowdsourcing through an unsupervised expertise estimation approach. *Decision Support Systems, 122*, 113065.

Moayedikia, A., Yeoh, W., Ong, K. L., & Boo, Y. L. (2020). Framework and literature analysis for crowdsourcing's answer aggregation. *Journal of Computer Information Systems, 60*(1), 49–60.

Morschheuser, B., & Hamari, J. (2019). The gamification of work: Lessons from crowdsourcing. *Journal of Management Inquiry, 28*(2), 145–148.

Murillo-Zamorano, L. R., Sánchez, J. Á. L., & Muñoz, C. B. (2020). Gamified crowdsourcing in higher education: A theoretical framework and a case study. *Thinking Skills and Creativity, 36*, 100645.

Neto, F. R. A., & Santos, C. A. (2018). Understanding crowdsourcing projects: A systematic review of tendencies, workflow, and quality management. *Information Processing & Management, 54*(4), 490–506.

Niu, X. J., Qin, S. F., Vines, J., Wong, R., & Lu, H. (2019). Key crowdsourcing technologies for product design and development. *International Journal of Automation and Computing, 16*(1), 1–15.

Niu, X. J., Qin, S. F., Zhang, H., Wang, M., & Wong, R. (2018). Exploring product design quality control and assurance under both traditional and crowdsourcing-based design environments. *Advances in Mechanical Engineering, 10*(12), 1–23.

Paik, J. H., Scholl, M., Sergeev, R., Randazzo, S., & Lakhani, K. R. (2020). Innovation contests for high-tech procurement. *Research-Technology Management, 63*(2), 36–45.

Papangelis, K., Potena, D., Smari, W. W., Storti, E., & Wu, K. (2019). Advanced technologies and systems for collaboration and computer supported cooperative work. *Future Generation Computer Systems, 95*, 764–774.

Pee, L. G., Koh, E., & Goh, M. (2018). Trait motivations of crowdsourcing and task choice: A distal-proximal perspective. *International Journal of Information Management, 40*, 28–41.

Phuttharak, J., & Loke, S. (2020). Exploring incentive mechanisms for mobile crowdsourcing: Sense of safety in a Thai city. *International Journal of Urban Sciences, 24*(1), 13–34.

Piezunka, H., & Dahlander, L. (2019). Idea rejected, tie formed: Organizations' feedback on crowdsourced ideas. *Academy of Management Journal, 62*(2), 503–530.

Pinto, J. M. G., El Maarry, K., & Balke, W. T. (2019). Fine-tuning gold questions in crowdsourcing tasks using probabilistic and siamese neural network models. *The Journal of Web Science, 6.*

Pohlisch, J. (2020). Internal open innovation-lessons learned from internal crowdsourcing at SAP. *Sustainability, 12*, 4245.

Pollok, P., Lüttgens, D., & Piller, F. T. (2019). Attracting solutions in crowdsourcing contests: The role of knowledge distance, identity disclosure, and seeker status. *Research Policy, 48*(1), 98–114.

Pulay, A., & Asino, T. I. (2019). An exploratory study examining group dynamics in a Hackathon. *International Journal of Virtual and Augmented Reality (IJVAR), 3*(2), 1–10.

Renard, D., & Davis, J. G. (2019). Social interdependence on crowdsourcing platforms. *Journal of Business Research, 103*, 186–194.

Rowledge, L. R. (2019). *Crowdrising: Building a sustainable world through mass collaboration.* London: Routledge.

Saab, F., Elhajj, I. H., Kayssi, A., & Chehab, A. (2019). Modelling cognitive bias in crowdsourcing systems. *Cognitive Systems Research, 58*, 1–18.

Sari, A., Tosun, A., & Alptekin, G. I. (2019). A systematic literature review on crowdsourcing in software engineering. *Journal of Systems and Software, 153*, 200–219.

Schäfer, S., Antons, D., Lüttgens, D., Piller, F., & Salge, T. O. (2017). Talk to your crowd: Principles for effective communication in crowdsourcing a few key principles for communicating with solvers can help contest sponsors maintain and grow their base of participants. *Research-Technology Management, 60*(4), 33–42.

Schenk, E., Guittard, C., & Pénin, J. (2019). Open or proprietary? Choosing the right crowdsourcing platform for innovation. *Technological Forecasting and Social Change, 144*, 303–310.

Schlagwein, D., Cecez-Kecmanovic, D., & Hanckel, B. (2019). Ethical norms and issues in crowdsourcing practices: A Habermasian analysis. *Information Systems Journal, 29*(4), 811–837.

Segev, E. (2020). Crowdsourcing contests. *European Journal of Operational Research, 281*(2), 241–255.

Sheehan, K. B., & Pittman, M. (2019). Straight from the source? Media framing of creative crowd labor and resultant ethical concerns. *Journal of Business Ethics, 154*(2), 575–585.

Shergadwala, M., Forbes, H., Schaefer, D., & Panchal, J. H. (2020). Challenges and research directions in crowdsourcing for engineering design: An interview study with industry professionals. *IEEE Transactions on Engineering Management.* DOI: 10.1109/TEM.2020.2983551

Shi, P., Wang, W., Zhou, Y., Jiang, J., Jiang, Y., Hao, Z., & Yu, J. (2019). Practical POMDP-based test mechanism for quality assurance in volunteer crowdsourcing. *Enterprise Information Systems, 13*(7–8), 979–1001.

Si, Y., Wu, H., & Liu, Q. (2020). Factors influencing doctors' participation in the provision of medical services through crowdsourced health care information websites: Elaboration-likelihood perspective study. *JMIR Medical Informatics, 8*(6), e16704.

Soliman, W., & Tuunainen, V. K. (2015). Understanding continued use of crowdsourcing systems: An interpretive study. *Journal of Theoretical and Applied Electronic Commerce Research, 10*(1), 1–18.

Song, Z., Zhang, H., & Dolan, C. (2020). Promoting disaster resilience: Operation mechanisms and self-organizing processes of crowdsourcing. *Sustainability, 12*(5), 1862.

Soon, J. M., & Saguy, I. S. (2017). Crowdsourcing: A new conceptual view for food safety and quality. *Trends in Food Science & Technology, 66*, 63–72.

Suzuki, Y., Matsuda, Y., & Nakamura, S. (2019). Additional operations of simple HITs on microtask crowdsourcing for worker quality prediction. *Journal of Information Processing, 27*, 51–60.

Tang, W., Wei, C., Cao, B., Wu, D., Li, K. T., Lu, H., . . . Mollan, K. R. (2018). Crowdsourcing to expand HIV testing among men who have sex with men in China: A closed cohort stepped wedge cluster randomized controlled trial. *PLoS Medicine, 15*(8), e1002645.

Tekic, A., & Willoughby, K. W. (2020). Configuring intellectual property management strategies in co-creation: A contextual perspective. *Innovation, 22*(2), 128–159.

Thuan, N. H., Antunes, P., & Johnstone, D. (2016). Factors influencing the decision to crowdsource: A systematic literature review. *Information Systems Frontiers, 18*(1), 47–68.

Thuan, N. H., Antunes, P., & Johnstone, D. (2017). A process model for establishing business process crowdsourcing. *Australasian Journal of Information Systems, 21*, 1–21.

Tong, Y., Zhou, Z., Zeng, Y., Chen, L., & Shahabi, C. (2020). Spatial crowdsourcing: A survey. *VLDB Journal, 29*(1), 217–250.

Torfing, J., Sørensen, E., & Røiseland, A. (2019). Transforming the public sector into an arena for co-creation: Barriers, drivers, benefits, and ways forward. *Administration & Society, 51*(5), 795–825.

Troll, J., Blohm, I., & Leimeister, J. M. (2019). Why incorporating a platform-intermediary can increase crowdsourcees' engagement. *Business & Information Systems Engineering, 61*(4), 433–450.

Tucker, J. D., Tang, W., Li, H., Liu, C., Fu, R., Tang, S., . . . Tangthanasup, T. M. (2018). Crowdsourcing designathon: A new model for multisectoral collaboration. *BMJ Innovations, 4*(2), 46–50.

Urra, O., & Ilarri, S. (2019). Spatial crowdsourcing with mobile agents in vehicular networks. *Vehicular Communications, 17*, 10–34.

Van Galen, C. W. (2019). Creating an audience: Experiences from the Surinamese slave registers crowdsourcing project. *Historical Methods: A Journal of Quantitative and Interdisciplinary History, 52*(3), 178–194.

Vianna, F. R. P. M., Graeml, A. R., & Peinado, J. (2020). The role of crowdsourcing in industry 4.0: A systematic literature review. *International Journal of Computer Integrated Manufacturing, 33*(4), 411–427.

Wang, G., & Yu, L. (2019). The game equilibrium of scientific crowdsourcing solvers based on the hotelling model. *Journal of Open Innovation: Technology, Market, and Complexity, 5*(4), 89.

Wang, G., & Yu, L. (2020). Analysis of enterprise sustainable crowdsourcing incentive mechanism based on principal-agent model. *Sustainability, 12*(8), 3238.

Wang, M. M., Wang, J. J., & Zhang, W. N. (2019). How to enhance solvers' continuance intention in crowdsourcing contest. *Online Information Review, 44*(1), 238–257.

Wang, Z., Hu, J., Lv, R., Wei, J., Wang, Q., Yang, D., & Qi, H. (2018). Personalized privacy-preserving task allocation for mobile crowdsensing. *IEEE Transactions on Mobile Computing, 18*(6), 1330–1341.

Wehn, U., & Almomani, A. (2019). Incentives and barriers for participation in community-based environmental monitoring and information systems: A critical analysis and integration of the literature. *Environmental Science & Policy, 101*, 341–357.

Wen, Z., & Lin, L. (2016). Optimal fee structures of crowdsourcing platforms. *Decision Sciences, 47*(5), 820–850.

Wilson, M., Robson, K., & Botha, E. (2017). Crowdsourcing in a time of empowered stakeholders: Lessons from crowdsourcing campaigns. *Business Horizons, 60*(2), 247–253.

Xia, H., & McKernan, B. (2020). Privacy in crowdsourcing: A review of the threats and challenges. *Computer Supported Cooperative Work (CSCW), 29*, 263–301.

Xiao, L., & Ke, T. (2019). The influence of platform incentives on actual carriers' continuous participation intention of non-vehicle operating carrier platform. *Asia Pacific Journal of Marketing and Logistics, 31*(5), 1269–1286.

Yang, K. (2019). Research on factors affecting solvers' participation time in online crowdsourcing contests. *Future Internet, 11*(8), 176.

Ye, H. J., & Kankanhalli, A. (2017). Solvers' participation in crowdsourcing platforms: Examining the impacts of trust, and benefit and cost factors. *The Journal of Strategic Information Systems, 26*(2), 101–117.

Yuan, S. T. D., & Hsieh, C. F. (2018). An impactful crowdsourcing intermediary design- a case of a service imagery crowdsourcing system. *Information Systems Frontiers, 20*(4), 841–862.

Zhang, S., Singh, P. V., & Ghose, A. (2019). A structural analysis of the role of superstars in crowdsourcing contests. *Information Systems Research, 30*(1), 15–33.

3 Crowdsourcing during the COVID-19 crisis

3.1 Crowdsourcing in previous crises

One of the main applications of crowdsourcing in crisis is the collection of information about what happened almost immediately. This facilitates the development of responses to the event (Hassan & Rahim, 2017). When a location is attached to these data, it is called mapping. Specifically, crowdsourced crisis mapping is defined as "the provision of services by an international and/or online community, who gather, analyze and map critical information related to disaster-affected populations" (Hunt & Specht, 2019, p. 1).

One of the most well-known examples of this is Ushahidi,[1] a nonprofit platform created to identify on the map the places where violent actions took place after the elections in Kenya in 2008. Since its foundation, numerous crowdsourcing projects have used it as a base. Among them are several focused on crisis management. For example, Ushahidi was very helpful in locating where help was needed after the Haiti earthquake in 2010 (Norheim-Hagtun & Meier, 2010) and after Hurricane Irma in Miami in 2017 (Anthony, 2018).

Moreover, Ushahidi has collaborated with the Center for Excellence in Disaster Management and Humanitarian Assistance, the US agency for promoting disaster preparedness and social resilience in Asia and the Pacific, to create a crowdsourcing platform for this region only. This is the Crisis Preparedness Platform. This decision was motivated by the large number of natural disasters that occur in the area. The affected population informs about an event through the platform. The platform aggregates these data and displays them on a map, facilitating the effectiveness and speed of response (Ushahidi, n.d.).

Another crowdsourcing platform for performance during crisis is Peta-Bencana,[2] formerly called PetaJakarta. It was created in 2013 to address the damage caused by the floods in Jakarta (Indonesia). On this platform,

DOI: 10.4324/9781003290872-3

volunteers send information about disasters in real time and point out their location. In this way, the population, authorities, and emergency teams in the area can make better decisions.

Calls have also been made for help in crises not caused by natural disasters. For example, Malaysia Airlines flight 370 disappeared in 2014, and eight million people collaborated in its search for months analyzing images (Poblet et al., 2018). Finally, it is worth noting the important role played by social networks in this context, not only to seek the support of other individuals who are going through the same situation but also as a basis for the organization and implementation of responses born from citizenship itself (Pyle et al., 2019).

3.2 COVID context

At the beginning of January 2020, several cases of pneumonia of unknown origin were detected in Wuhan (China). They seem to be related to a market of fish and live animals, suggesting a link between this disease and exposure to animals. While pneumonia is a common disease at that time of year, the fact that 44 patients were admitted on January 3 and 11 of them were in serious condition raise the alarm (WHO, 2020a).

The Chinese authorities announced on January 9 that the cause of this pneumonia was a new type of coronavirus different from those previously known in humans. The knowledge available to date suggested that the virus was not transmitted in a significant way between people. In view of the need for further research, the following day, the WHO recommended that precautionary measures be taken, such as avoiding direct contact with infected people and hand washing to prevent spread (WHO, 2020b). During the following days, the WHO offered different documents to guide countries about the management of the new disease and notified the public about the first cases outside China, specifically, in Thailand and Japan. A week later, cases of coronavirus infection were detected in the United States and France. The disease had reached America and Europe (WHO, 2020c).

As of January 30, one month after the WHO learned of the existence of pneumonia of unknown origin, there were 98 confirmed cases in 18 countries outside China. In eight of them, contagion had occurred among people not connected with China. This caused the WHO to declare that the new coronavirus represented a Public Health Emergency of International Concern (WHO, 2020d). The number of infections soared during the following weeks, and on March 11, 2020, WHO Director General Tedros Adhanom declared in a press conference that COVID-19 was considered a pandemic (WHO, 2020e).

The main measures taken by most countries to stop the spread of the coronavirus have been movement restrictions and home confinement. This has meant great changes in daily life. Educational centers and establishments selling nonessential goods have been closed, and most activities have been transferred to the digital plane (Weil & Murugesan, 2020). In this context, the possibilities offered by crowdsourcing have been used to support the fight against the effects of the virus and facilitate the return to normality. The following are the defining characteristics of the essential elements of the activities that have been carried out during the months after the declaration of a pandemic. The section also lists and discusses some factors that may have facilitated their development, as well as others that may have hindered it.

3.3 Crowdsourcing elements

3.3.1 Crowdsourcer

Public institutions, companies, nonprofit organizations, and citizen associations have launched calls within the framework of the pandemic. Crowdsourcing may represent an alternative for public institutions to achieve citizen engagement during the COVID-19 crisis. According to the study by Chen et al. (2020), the promotion of dialogue by governments through social networks increases the commitment of the population in the context of COVID-19. Citizens perceive their interest and feel valued and recognized. This is similar to soliciting opinions or ideas through a crowdsourcing call. Such a call can be crucial for facing this crisis in countries where the level of commitment within the society is low.

On the other hand, some of the social projects launched by these entities are created and organized by the citizens themselves. This usually occurs when a group of the population believes that some of its collective needs are not being met by the authorities (Komninos, 2019). In the context of COVID-19, the government has not been able to meet all the challenges it faces. Therefore, citizen crowdsourcing projects have emerged to support the community members themselves.

Solutions are born from a single individual or from citizen networks to compensate for the sudden absence of food or basic necessities. In this situation, informal organizations have grown rapidly and facilitated supply by working, generally, independently from institutions (Calori & Federici, 2020). It should be noted that, in the context of COVID-19, individuals who have created content related to it have attracted the attention of a larger audience than many reputable specialized websites thanks to social networks (Pérez-Escoda et al., 2020). Likewise, some companies have executed actions within their social responsibility strategy to help the community in this period (Ebrahim & Buheji, 2020). Others have supported and collaborated with other agents to launch calls for proposals.

3.3.2 Platform

To carry out the activities, the crowdsourcers have used both open and proprietary platforms. Two types of open platforms that have been of great help during this period are collaborative maps and the sites that collect technical challenges. An example of the former is Ushahidi. As in other crisis, it has been used to pinpoint different locations, from stores that have extended their hours or provide assistance to people in need.

With regard to technical challenges, one of the advantages offered by these platforms is that they already have a community of regular users who contribute to projects on a relatively frequent basis. An example is InnoCentive,[3] one of the most popular websites that raise innovation issues proposed by different crowdsourcers. During the beginning of the pandemic, it hosted several issues related to COVID-19. Social networks have also been used to develop crowdsourcing projects during this period. For example, Sun et al. (2020) collected data to analyze the effects of the coronavirus through a Chinese social network targeting healthcare workers. The advantage of social networks is the large number of users who access them.

3.3.3 Task

Poblet et al. (2018) examine the use of crowdsourcing during emergencies and divide participants into the following categories based on the task they perform:

- Sensors: These actors send raw data, which can be collected by the functionalities of the device used for participation or entered manually by each individual.
- Social computers: They communicate through social networks, and from there, the content that is analyzed is obtained.
- Reporters: They also intervene through social networks. However, unlike individuals in the previous category, they offer first-hand, real-time information about the event that has taken place. In addition, they usually contain metadata such as hashtags, which facilitates subsequent processing.

- Microtaskers: These actors perform slightly more complex tasks, such as tagging images or adding coordinates.

Poblet et al. (2018) focus on microtasks related to data generation and processing, which are very useful in managing crisis. However, more complex tasks are needed to address COVID-19. The magnitude of this crisis requires great solutions. These macrotasks can be technical or creative or a combination of both. For example, creating designs for medical equipment can facilitate health care during this period. Additionally, the contributions of the crowd are added depending on the characteristics of the project. In the previous case, a single proposal is the solution to the challenge posed. On the other hand, if crowdsourcing is used to collect data and carry out scientific studies regarding coronavirus, the contributions are aggregated.

3.3.4 Participants

With regard to the skills of the crowd, platforms call for the participation of people in two main categories: people with certain qualifications and the whole population. In the first category are the calls directed to researchers, health workers, or engineers, among others. These are activities that require certain skills or knowledge to participate. They propose, for example, creating designs of medical equipment to improve health care or collaborating in the scientific study of the virus. Not all citizens are able to collaborate in these projects.

Second, in this context where any help is welcome, many calls open participation to the whole population. Ratner et al. (2020) reflect on the lessons we have learned during the first stage of the pandemic. Referring to the health field, they propose facilitating collaboration among all parties, patients, health workers, and community members to foster knowledge sharing, learning, and creative problem-solving. Moreover, they point out that the agents who are used to working with few resources should be heard. While reputable professionals in specialized centers that excel in their sector have much knowledge that they can apply to the fight against COVID-19, those who often work with limitations are better able to come up with creative solutions.

Some of the typologies of crowdsourcing that were developed during this period and promote the participation of the entire population are citizen support networks and crowdfunding. To intervene in these types, it is not necessary to possess any specific skill. Crowdsourcing aims at collaboration between individuals in performing small tasks and is based on the altruism of the community (Peng, 2017). Crowdfunding, on the other hand, encourages monetary donations to finance a given project. Both of these typologies can be adapted to the conditions of the pandemic and help curb its effects through the collaboration of any individual.

It should also be remembered that these efforts can be initiated by any entity or individual, even by large institutions that have never asked for donations before. This is the case of the World Health Organization, which in March launched a crowdfunding campaign to finance the response to the virus. In just 10 days, it raised 71 million dollars through the altruism of 170,000 individuals and organizations, including Facebook and Google (Usher, 2020).

However, although crowdsourcing activities are usually directed at only one of these groups, there are large projects that launch simultaneous calls to the entire population and to a specific group within it. One example during the pandemic is COVID Moonshot,[4] which aims to promote the development of a coronavirus antiviral treatment. Moonshot proposes three tasks. Two can be done by any individual, and one can be done only by those with particular skills and knowledge. The latter group is asked to develop and submit antiviral designs or data from experiments in this regard. All contributions are published on the website. In this way, the exchange and generation of new ideas are encouraged.

On the other hand, Moonshot asks the general public for donations to manufacture and test the most promising designs. This campaign is advertised on the website but takes place through GoFundMe,[5] a major crowdfunding platform. It also urges participants to share their computers' processing capability in order to run molecular simulations. Similarly, COVID Moonshot makes this call visible on its website, but the activity takes place on Folding@home,[6] a distributed computing platform. This task is passive. That is, the participants only have to agree to share their resources, but they do not actively carry out any work.

These activities are complementary. They all help achieve a common goal: to accelerate the development of an antiviral treatment against the new coronavirus. The possibility of carrying out several tasks within the same project, only some of which require specific skills, is not common. In fact, COVID Moonshot defines itself as ambitious.

3.4 Favorable conditions for crowdsourcing

3.4.1 Motivated participants

The COVID-19 crisis affected the entire population. Regardless of whether one has suffered from the disease, we have all suffered its consequences. Closure of stores and educational centers, home confinement. . . .

One may think that one of the motivations for participating in crowd-sourcing in this context is to help alleviate the effects of the pandemic and overcome it more quickly. In this way, society as a whole benefits, including the person who participates.

For example, being a victim is a motivating condition for collaboration. According to the study by Yardley et al. (2018), having been a victim of a crime and feeling that a case is similar are two of the main incentives for participating in calls urging citizens to collaborate in the resolution of crimes. Riccardi (2016) analyzes the use of crowdsourcing as a disaster response. He notes that a key motivation among those affected to participate is the desire to take some control over the situation. Crowdsourcing situations cause confusion, and human nature has the impulse to try to control events.

Both self-interest and the willingness to benefit other individuals act as motivators in crowdsourcing (Alam et al., 2020). Selfishness, the desire to help the group to which the individual belongs, the feeling of belonging to the cause, and pure altruism represent incentives (Alam et al., 2020; John-Matthews et al., 2020; Luo et al., 2017). In the context of COVID-19, it is difficult to distinguish which of these motivations drives participants. All individuals and their loved ones are potential patients of the disease. In addition, helping in the fight against the coronavirus helps society as a whole as well as individuals and their loved ones.

On the other hand, it should be noted that although monetary rewards are the most recurrent incentive in crowdsourcing, they are not necessary (Komninos, 2019). Moreover, in the context of the pandemic, they may not have the desired effect. According to the study by Kim et al. (2019), financial rewards do not act as a motivating element for users of a healthcare volunteer platform. Ogie et al. (2019) advise against the use of monetary incentives for crowdsourcing activities during emergencies. These authors argue that, under these circumstances, payments are contrary to the voluntary nature of the project itself. Ideally, the crowd should only participate in an altruistic way to counteract the negative effects of the crisis and to encourage the return of the community to normality. Likewise, the study by Cappa et al. (2019b) shows that the possibility of achieving a benefit for society significantly increases the number of contributions received in crowdsourcing. According to these authors, incentives that support social causes can act as a motivating element for participants and thus improve the results of these experiences.

It can be said that the desire to help others is what motivates the members of citizen collaboration networks during the coronavirus crisis. In these cases, no financial compensation is offered, and the identity of those who help is not published. Participants do such work out of altruism, trying to alleviate the effects the pandemic is having on others. However, in other projects in this context, monetary incentives are recommended.

Another option during a pandemic is to draw on a community already in existence. One example is the activity launched by the University of Chicago: UChicago Crowdsourcing COVID-19 History Project. This is a call to all those who are connected to it, such as students, families, and workers. The aim is to collect videos, images, audio, or texts describing their experience during the coronavirus crisis. With this material, the project intends to produce a documentary or an exhibition that will serve as a legacy for future generations to learn about the experiences of people living in this period of time (University of Chicago, 2020). In this case, participation is restricted, but the level of collaboration may be high as a result of the feeling of belonging to the community. On the one hand, the group has a connection with the requester. On the other hand, the project represents an opportunity to feel connected with other individuals in a moment of social distancing.

As mentioned earlier, any entity or individual can act as a crowdsourcer in crowdsourcing. During the pandemic, even well-known artists chose this tool. On May 1, singer Justin Bieber made a call through his Instagram profile to ask his fans to help him create the video clip of his new song with Ariana Grande (Bieber, 2020). The call was aimed at the entire population, although he made special mention of the students who should have graduated during the confinement. To participate, they could post on social networks a video of themselves dancing inside their home and, if possible, wearing the outfit they would have worn to the ceremony, accompanied by a hashtag with the title of the musical theme. Only one week later, Ariana Grande announced the premiere of the video clip on the same social network (Grande, 2020a).

Several motivational elements can be identified in this call. First, participating means collaborating with your idol. This, in itself, can be a sufficient incentive to send a contribution. In addition, appearing in the music video can generate reputation and recognition. The video is available on platforms such as YouTube and has millions of views (Grande, 2020b), such that millions of people have seen the participants on screen. Finally, this project supports a social cause. The profits from this song were donated to the First Responders Children's Foundation, which would pass on the funds to the children of those who have worked on the front lines of the coronavirus in the form of grants and scholarships. That is, this call combines selfish and altruistic motivations for participation.

Developing solutions to a technical problem requires skills and time. This is usually rewarded in an economic way. An example of this is the challenges launched through InnoCentive,[7] one of the most well-known open crowdsourcing platforms. In it, the crowdsourcers pose challenges and establish a prize for the winning proposal. During the pandemic, an exclusive section for calls related to the coronavirus has been created, offering financial prizes for the best contributions (InnoCentive, 2020).

One of the arguments supporting the decision to keep these prizes is set out below. Acar (2019) analyzes the relationship between the motivation of the participants and the adequacy of their contributions compared to the requirements set by the call. Receiving contributions that meet the established conditions is of the utmost importance in projects that request the submission of proposals that solve a complex problem. In these cases, the contributions must be evaluated individually to check their suitability and identify which is the most appropriate. The more contributions there are, the longer it takes to evaluate them. If many of them do not meet the requirements, this is a waste of time. Investing more resources decreases the efficiency of crowdsourcing. In addition, during the onset of the pandemic, solutions needed to be found urgently. This is especially the case regarding technical problems, such as those addressed by InnoCentive, which sought ideas for new designs of effective coronavirus protection and masks, among others.

Acar (2019) hypothesizes that prosocial motivation, focused on performing an activity to benefit others, is positively related to the appropriateness of contributions in crowdsourcing. However, the author finds this relationship to be negative. Therefore, the degree of fit between the contributions received and the requirements requested during the pandemic may be low. This implies a greater effort in evaluation and screening, leading to an increase in the time needed to decide which solution is most appropriate. At such a time, no time can be wasted, and proposals need to be in line with the call. Therefore, relying on altruism as a motivating element does not seem to be an adequate option.

However, there are exceptions to this, and these complex tasks can be accomplished voluntarily without the possibility of achieving a prize. An example is the case of Ennomotive.[8] This is a platform aimed at engineers that works in a similar way to InnoCentive. In the context of COVID-19, the platform has launched a challenge to obtain designs of respirators to help patients with the disease (Ennomotive, 2020). The crowdsourcer is the platform itself, whose team has joined the fight. In terms of activity, the platform clearly indicates that it does not offer any prize in exchange for participation. However, the first phase of the call has been a success, and a second phase has been created to ask the crowd for ideas to improve the design selected in the previous phase.

3.4.2 Time to participate

The lack of time is one of the main reasons people do not participate in or abandon a crowdsourcing project (Wehn & Almomani, 2019). Moreover, according to the study by Kim et al. (2019), time spent on the task is the main barrier users state to answer why they do not participate in a digital volunteer activity. Individuals may have little free time in their daily lives. However, this has changed due to the coronavirus. Measures to contain its spread have meant that one can only leave home to carry out essential activities, such as working if there is no possibility of doing so from home or going to buy food and medicine. In this context, most people have available all the time they used to spend on leisure and work outside the home.

Likewise, the sadness and boredom resulting from this situation has encouraged the population to experience a slowdown in time (Droit-Volet et al., 2020). According to Ogden (2020), this distortion in time perception is related to the degree of satisfaction of an individual with his or her level of social interaction. Specifically, the more dissatisfied an individual is, the slower it seems that time passes during confinement, and vice versa. In this context, crowdsourcing is a tool that can facilitate avoidance and promote the faster passage of time. Focusing attention on this activity can prevent boredom. In addition, some projects allow contact with other participants, which can improve satisfaction regarding the degree of social interaction. In this way, participating in an activity can help make the period of confinement more enjoyable and reduce its perceived duration.

Moreover, depression and anxiety are common among the population as a result of confinement (Fullana et al., 2020). To confront this issue, Chew et al. (2020) recommend encouraging different behaviors. Among them are the realization of online play activities to improve skills and encourage digital support groups. Some users claim to participate in crowdsourcing for the fun and intellectual stimulation it provides (Bakici, 2020). Another motivation for participating in crowdsourcing is to feel productive during free time (Deng & Joshi, 2016). Finally, some people have decided to take advantage of this increased free time to develop new skills or try new entertainment alternatives (Mackolil & Mackolil, 2020). This can also be obtained through crowdsourcing, since one of the incentives it offers is the possibility of learning (Ghezzi et al., 2018).

3.4.3 Ease of dissemination

For an individual to participate effectively, not only must he be motivated and have sufficient skills to carry out the task, but there must also be a trigger that moves him to do so (Chen, 2019). Therefore, efforts have to be dedicated to the dissemination of a call. It is impossible to anticipate a crisis, a disaster, or an emergency. This reduces the time to plan a crowdsourcing activity as a response, which makes it difficult to organize. Similar to the planning and design phase, the communication of a project during COVID-19 must be carried out quickly and effectively. The aim is to reach a large number of people and to successfully motivate a high percentage of them to participate. Attracting collaborators is an essential aspect for a project to develop (Hannewijk et al., 2020). During the pandemic, several factors have facilitated this.

First, the media have focused on reporting on the evolution of the pandemic, prevention measures, scientific advances about the new coronavirus, and its effect on society and the economy (Haroon & Rizvi, 2020; Liu et al., 2020). Politicians have had to devote all their efforts to contain and fight the effects of COVID-19, and confinement has led to the cancellation of all kinds of events. In short, the media can only report on the coronavirus. Some media have highlighted crowdsourcing projects, favoring their dissemination. For example, the *New York Times* published a news story about the COVID Symptom Study app, a crowdsourcing-based application that asks users for information about their symptoms to carry out scientific research (Jacobs, 2020), and another news story about a Facebook call for designs for healthcare material to treat COVID-19 (Petri, 2020). The *Washington Post* echoed several calls for donations of protective equipment (Chason, 2020). These media outlets have a large audience. Giving visibility to them helps involve a greater percentage of the population, as individuals become aware of the them and decide to participate. In addition, appearing in the media brings credibility to a project (Ogie et al., 2019).

On the other hand, crowdsourcing can be supported by social networks to have a greater scope (Ilmi et al., 2020). The public is familiar with the use of social networks, and implementing a strategy through this medium is low cost for the organizer. Therefore, social networks offer a good alternative to access the knowledge and experience of the crowd (Candi et al., 2018). It should be noted that companies can analyze the opinions that users pour into the networks and include their vision within the innovation process to create products and services adapted to what the public wants (Patroni et al., 2020). However, this cannot be considered crowdsourcing since there is no call from the organizer and no task has been set.

Social networks can offer a scenario where the activity takes place and provide their communication strategy. Crowdsourcing announcements on social networks have a greater chance of being seen the more time users spend on them. Their use has increased due to COVID-19. According to the study by Rodriguez-Rey et al. (2020), activities related to contact with other individuals are the ones that have been carried out the most during confinement in Spain. Specifically, 85.2% of respondents used social networks or shared content on them. This has also happened in other countries. For example, in China, more than one-third of the participants in the research of Ni et al. (2020) used social networks for at least two hours a day. Other studies have shown increased time spent using social networks and digital media during confinement in Italy (Cellini et al., 2020) and India (Sinha et al., 2020).

This increase in usage time positively affects crowdsourcing, as it helps disseminate the projects. However, it is worth noting that only a small percentage of Internet users who are aware of the existence of an activity decide to participate in it. Even so, if the number of people who have found out about the project is very high, it can be said that the number of potential participants is also high.

Both the media and social networks act as loudspeakers for calls. However, there is another factor that also encourages participation and is of great relevance. This is social influence, which refers to an individual's perception that people who are important to him and whose opinion he values think he should be involved in a project (Wang et al., 2020). According to the study by Nor et al. (2019), social influence plays an important role in attracting collaborators. Most of the participants in their research stated that they had accessed a virtual volunteer community because they had been invited by friends or a superior.

Moreover, Yaseen and Al Omoush (2020) state that social influence affects the intention to participate in a crowdsourcing project when it takes place in a time of crisis. In this sense, Havas et al. (2017) highlight the unpredictable nature of the crowd that participates in a crowdsourcing activity to cope with an emergency. These authors propose a series of measures to facilitate citizen collaboration in these circumstances. Among them are the creation and maintenance of a small group of volunteers who are committed and prepared to recruit participants when a crisis occurs. This can be done when the existence of a threat is known in advance. However, the situation arising from COVID-19 could not be foreseen. Even so, efforts can be made during the early stages of planning and designing a crowdsourcing project related to the new coronavirus to recruit participants who will later release the call. In addition, its reach can be increased through social networks.

Some calls have encouraged this process of social influence and encouraged the participants to attract more people. One of these is the COVID-19 Campaign Survey, a project launched by the United Nations

Human Settlements Programme (UN-Habitat). It consists of a question-naire to learn about the situation and the effects of COVID-19 in urban areas. The call has a global character and is addressed to all individuals. A badge is offered when a participant completes the survey. The website of the project states that "you can post [it] to your social media account. The badge will show your friends that you helped UN-Habitat in this data collection initiative-and will serve to motivate them to help, too" (UN-Habitat, 2020). UN-Habitat pursues a dual objective through this strategy. On the one hand, it serves as a reputation mechanism. This recognition signals which users have collaborated and sets them apart from the rest. On the other hand, it works as a communication element. The individuals who share it through social networks to let their contacts know that they have contributed also give publicity to it. In this way, each user can attract more participants. If this reputation system functions correctly, the individuals who find out about the call by publishing the merit of a close friend in social networks may also participate. Thus, the aim is to attract a large volume of participants so that the results of the survey are reliable.

3.4.4 Crowdsourcer's experience

Having experience implies having previously faced something. As in any field, experience positively affects the viability of a crowdsourcing project (Thuan et al., 2016). It is a factor that favors its success, and the risk a crowdsourcer runs when creating an activity decreases if it has developed another one previously (Blohm et al., 2018). In some cases, experienced crowdsourcers have used their knowledge to create new projects in the context of the pandemic.

For example, an increasing number of countries have open gov-ernment platforms that allow interaction with citizens. They rely on crowdsourcing to gather ideas and obtain the population's point of view on different issues. Several governments have taken advantage of these platforms to include challenges related to the fight against COVID-19. One such government is that of Brazil, whose National School of Public Administration manages the Desafíos platform,[9] a virtual space where citizens can participate in contests and propose solutions to public problems. During the pandemic, the platform launched challenges to improve the efficiency of the health system and mitigate the economic effects of the crisis. In return, it offers monetary rewards for winning solutions.

Another entity that has experience in these projects is NASA. This insti-tution focuses on innovation and makes frequent use of crowdsourcing.

The platform it uses is NASA@WORK (NASA, 2020a), to which only its workers have access. This type of crowdsourcing is called internal crowdsourcing (Malhotra et al., 2020). During the pandemic, NASA employees were invited to contribute ideas within this platform to address the shortage of personal protective equipment and respirators, as well as to find mechanisms to predict the evolution and effects of the new coronavirus (NASA, 2020b). However, NASA also launched another call aimed at the entire population. This is the NASA Space Apps COVID-19 Challenge,[10] which took place on May 30 and 31, 2020, in the form of a hackathon. This digital event brought together more than 15,000 participants from 150 countries.

Moreover, there are alternatives to facilitate the success of a call if the crowdsourcer does not have experience with crowdsourcing. One of them is to create an alliance with another entity that does have experience. The Lithuanian government collaborated with companies to develop HACK THE CRISIS,[11] a crowdsourcing event held between March 20 and 22 to collect proposals for both challenges and solutions. Among these companies is Garage48,[12] a company specialized in organizing hackathons. Garage48 contributed its knowledge to the project, making it easier to carry it out properly.

An open crowdsourcing platform can also be used. These platforms base their business model on developing this type of activity. The crowdsourcers who choose to use them must fill in a series of fields that the platform itself indicates, which simplifies the design process. In addition, the platform a community of users who often participate in challenges. Therefore, the project is guaranteed to be known, even if there is no complementary communication strategy.

3.4.5 Open resources

Some crowdsourcing activities require participants to possess specific knowledge or skills to participate in them. This is the case mainly when the task is to develop technical solutions to a complex problem. In the context of the pandemic, crowdsourcing represents a powerful tool for reaching individuals from any corner of the globe who have the ability to assist in a highly challenging task.

However, the new coronavirus is a challenge for everyone since it is unknown how it behaves and what is the most effective way to deal with it. Even the most highly trained health professionals, engineers, and researchers do not know how to respond since there is no precedent. Crowdsourcing is useless if the task undertaken is so complex that no individual has the capacity to solve it. Therefore, it is essential that findings be shared and, in this way, advance the related knowledge so that other voices can offer their understanding and ideas about it.

In this sense, during the beginning of the pandemic, we witnessed a wave of collaboration and solidarity. Scientific publishers have not been left behind. Most of them are of restricted access. To read their publications, individuals must pay in advance or have a subscription. This is a barrier for those who have the ability to develop technical solutions to the coronavirus but cannot spend resources to learn about the advances in this regard. To make knowledge accessible to any individual, the main publishers have opened access to all their content related to COVID-19. Some of these are Elsevier, Springer, or Wiley (Song & Karako, 2020).

This is a favorable condition for crowdsourcing. If publications about coronavirus are not freely accessible, only the individuals with specific skills who can afford the scientific content will have sufficient mastery of the subject to be able to participate. However, with this measure, any trained individual can be prepared to fight the effects of the virus in a technical way.

In this sense, Havas et al. (2017) recommend organizing activities to train and improve the skills of future volunteers in response to a call framed in a moment of crisis. Time was pressing during the initial moments of this pandemic, and resources needed to be directed toward creating solutions rather than training participants. Free resources can fill that role by making it easier for participants to carry out these activities on their own.

3.4.6 No economic benefit for the crowdsourcer

Another aspect that can favor the success of a call is the fact that its organizer does not seek to obtain profits through it. According to Alam et al. (2020), people are more willing to collaborate in projects that do not seek economic benefit than in ones proposed by companies for commercial purposes. The crowd try to avoid the commodification of their work, preferring to contribute to a public good.

When the call is aimed at helping specific individuals, such as citizen networks to run daily activities, such as going to the supermarket or pharmacy so that a sick or vulnerable neighbor does not have to leave home, it is clear that the platform is not marketing with its goodwill. On the other hand, when the project is managed by a company or requests designs that are likely to be manufactured and sold in the future, the crowd may decide not to participate. Therefore, if that is not the purpose of the call, it must be clearly expressed in the terms.

This was done by the Ennomotive platform in the previously mentioned challenge regarding the design of respirators for patients with

COVID-19. In the description of the call, in addition to noting that no financial prizes were offered to participants, it was stated that all solutions received would be in the public domain. Moreover, it was stated that the company itself would finance the construction of the selected prototypes (Ennomotive, 2020). In this way, Ennomotive suggested that it sought the good of society and not its own profit. It did not take over the intellectual rights to the contributions, but these could be consulted by any individual to develop respirators to help in the fight against the coronavirus.

It should be noted that while there is no direct economic benefit, there may be an indirect benefit. In this as in other projects, the image of the crowdsourcer is improved when it is seen as an entity committed to society. Such activities can also generate publicity, making the crowdsourcer known to a greater number of people. These and other reasons may cause an increase in future profits.

There is also some controversy regarding the ethics surrounding crowdsourcing. Certain projects are controversial because they resemble a job but do not offer the same protection or remuneration that is traditionally given to employees (Sheehan & Pittman, 2019). In fact, some authors argue that if remuneration is not adequate, crowdsourcing may be a new form of labor exploitation (Standing & Standing, 2018). However, if the crowdsourcer pursues the good of society rather than enriching itself, this problem is avoided.

3.5 Crowdsourcing barriers

3.5.1 No time for planning

While time to participate benefits these activities, the absence of time to plan acts against them. Before publishing the call and allowing the crowd to participate, the call must be designed and configured. This involves making decisions about the task to be performed, how contributions will be processed or what will be offered in return (Thuan et al., 2017). This stage should be carried out with caution since the choices made will condition the rest of the process. For example, the degree of problem specification influences the number of participants who are attracted (Jiang et al., 2020), and the way the task is described affects the effort that individuals put into its execution (Yang, 2019) and the quality of the contributions (Hu et al., 2020).

In addition, thought must be given to how the contributions will be used later (Jespersen, 2018). If one does not keep in mind how they will be processed and how the objective of the call will be achieved through them, they may be useless. For example, if the project is created to collect data to carry out research, one must consider what analyses will be applied to the information received. To obtain value through the activity, not only must quality contributions be collected, but they also must be processed in an appropriate manner to achieve their purpose (Cappa et al., 2019). Another aspect that must be considered beforehand is whether the contributions will be aggregated. It is necessary to consider in the first case the method that will be used and, in the second case, the strategy that will be used to select the winning proposal among all those received. It is advisable to design these steps beforehand; otherwise, the evaluation phase will take longer. In this case, it takes longer to obtain a solution, and the costs of the activity increase (Christensen & Karlsson, 2019).

Moreover, the design phase represents one of the most important areas of study regarding the role of the crowdsourcer (Nevo & Kotlarsky, 2020). However, solutions were urgently needed during the beginning of the pandemic, regardless of its scope, to find new designs of health material and to translate texts or recruit volunteers for medical studies. These tasks needed to be carried out as soon as possible. Therefore, the planning phase of the projects could not be delayed without negatively affecting it.

3.5.2 Digital divide

Crowdsourcing bases its existence on the Internet. This is a barrier for individuals who do not have access to Internet. There may be groups of people who want to participate but are unable to do so. These are usually the elderly and those with a low level of digital skills (Gooch et al., 2020). De' et al. (2020) note that those without adequate Internet connections have been excluded during the pandemic. This is especially problematic when digital services fall within basic sectors, such as education and health care. Therefore, researchers and politicians have been asked to pay attention to the digital divide and try to minimize its adverse effects on the most vulnerable population. This equally affects the crowd in crowdsourcing. Consequently, mechanisms must be designed to reduce this negative impact and make it easier for as many people as possible to participate.

For example, Ludwig et al. (2017) recommend trying to ensure that all those affected by a crisis can contribute to these calls and combine them with offline actions. Tucker et al. (2018) also reflect on how the digital divide affects crowdsourcing. According to these authors, the calls that are disseminated through digital social media have a smaller scope given that a percentage of the population does not use them despite having an

Internet connection and therefore the capacity to participate. To avoid this, the authors recommend complementing the promotion of the project with face-to-face activities.

However, due to the widespread confinement during the pandemic, it is impossible to carry out such activities. Therefore, other strategies must be created to increase their scope. For example, the appearance of projects in traditional media, such as television and the written press, can be encouraged. Even so, participation can only be carried out through electronic devices with an Internet connection. Older individuals, those living in rural areas, and those with low incomes may be less able to understand or may have limited participation (Fagherazzi et al., 2020). As a result of the restrictions imposed by the pandemic, some groups will inevitably be excluded because they have to stay at home.

3.5.3 Cyberattacks

During the COVID-19 crisis, the number of cyberattacks has increased. According to data from INTERPOL (2020), 59% of the cyber threats that have taken place during this period consist of Internet scams and phishing,[13] mainly emails impersonating government and health authorities, both national and global. Financial support campaigns and requests for collaboration and fraudulent donations related to COVID-19 have also been detected. This can directly affect crowdsourcing. Cyber threats generate distrust among Internet users, who may decide not to participate in a call for fear that it will not be legitimate. Even if a project is endorsed by a prestigious institution, people may know that agencies, such as the WHO, were impersonated during the first months of the pandemic. In this way, the support of a recognized entity does not generate the confidence it should in the crowd. Moreover, 22% of cyber threats during the start of the health crisis correspond to the creation of malicious domains, increasing by more than 500% (INTERPOL, 2020).

This proliferation of websites pretending to belong to government agencies or consolidated companies can equally harm crowdsourcing projects that aim to fight the effects of the coronavirus. On the one hand, these activities are also susceptible to attack. On the other hand, decreased security in the digital environment can diminish the confidence of the crowd and discourage participation. Furthermore, trust in the platform on which it is carried out can be a key factor in the success of the event, as it acts as a mediator between the motivation of the crowd and the intention to participate (Martínez, 2017). As mentioned earlier, the population was motivated to contribute to projects focused on mitigating the effects of COVID-19. However, this may not be enough to make their participation effective if the website or application where the activity takes place does not generate trust. This directly affects the calls since fewer contributions are received and thus reduces the chances of success.

Therefore, mechanisms must be created to provide security to the process in order to build trust. In this context, strategies have been developed that, although not directly focused on crowdsourcing, have allowed the security of digital activities to be improved as a whole. Different organizations have developed such strategies to combat the increase in cyberattacks during this period. Some of them were created by large companies in the technology sector. For example, on March 17, Facebook, Google, LinkedIn, Microsoft, Reddit, Twitter, and YouTube published a joint industry statement through their social networks. They stated the following:

> We are working closely together on COVID-19 response efforts. We're helping millions of people stay connected while also jointly combating fraud and misinformation about the virus, elevating authoritative content on our platforms, and sharing critical updates in coordination with government healthcare agencies around the world. We invite other companies to join us as we work to keep our communities healthy and safe.
>
> (Facebook Newsroom, 2020)

Others, in contrast, emanate from citizens' associations. One example is the CTI League.[14] This is a community of volunteers created on March 14, 2020, to fight cyberattacks on strategic sectors in the context of the pandemic. Specifically, they are responsible for neutralizing and preventing these attacks, as well as supporting and monitoring cyberspace in the medical, emergency, and public health sectors. In just one month, the community managed to recruit over 1,400 members from 76 countries through crowdsourcing. To participate, individuals must have great skills and mastery in the field. Some of the volunteers are professionals with senior positions in large technology companies, such as Microsoft and Amazon (Menn, 2020). Thanks to their work, 2,833 threats were eliminated, and more than 2,000 weaknesses were detected in health institutions in that period. Among the targets of these attacks were the United Nations (UN) and the WHO.

These actions, although not expressly created by any crowdsourcer to facilitate its own project, benefit them. First, they combat and hinder the work of cybercriminals and create a secure environment for anyone operating over the Internet. Among them are crowdsourcers, platforms, and participants in crowdsourcing. Second, spreading news about the implementation of these strategies supports the creation of trust among the crowd. Thanks to them, the perception of risk linked to digital interactions can be reduced, which allows to eliminate possible obstacles to the intention to participate in crowdsourcing. However, the protection mechanisms of the platforms themselves must also be strengthened to ensure the privacy of users and to prevent their participation from being detrimental to them.

3.5.4 Sensitive data

One of the main measures taken to contain the pandemic is contact tracing. This activity can be done in two ways. First, it can be completed manually, through the work of people assigned and trained to do it. These individuals represent key actors in the new normal. They are in charge of identifying which people have had contact with an infected person and regularly follow them up to stop the transmission of the virus and reduce the risk of new infections (WHO, 2020f).

On the other hand, tracing can be carried out digitally through mobile applications. Cohen et al. (2020) differentiate two approaches:

(1) Centralized: employed by the governments of China, South Korea, and Taiwan. The authorities monitor population movements through digital tracing done mainly through the location of their cell phones.
(2) Decentralized or user-centered: each individual has the ability to decide whether to send notifications.

One of the premises of crowdsourcing is that participation must be voluntary. Therefore, applications governed by a centralized approach cannot be considered crowdsourcing, but others can be. The crowdsourcer is usually a public authority who asks the entire population of the territory to use the platform created in order to register which people they have had contact with. In addition, if a positive diagnosis of coronavirus is made, it must be notified through this platform. In this way, the application informs those who have had close contact with the subject that they may be infected.

However, the population is concerned about personal privacy and security (Dwivedi et al., 2020). Their data may be exposed, which represent a barrier to expanding the use of such applications. Therefore, strategies to build trust must be implemented. In this sense, Google and Apple have allied to develop a reliable technology to support these platforms (Google, 2020). This is an application programming interface (API) that can be used by organizations interested in controlling the spread of the virus through this method. This exposure notification API uses Bluetooth on participants' cell phones to send signals anonymously and register which other devices are nearby. In this way, the identity of the users is not made public. Authorities in many countries base their applications on it, for example, Immuni[15] in Italy, STAYAWAY COVID[16] in Portugal, and Corona-Warn-App in Germany.[17]

Another barrier refers to the legal level. With regard to sensitive data, the regulations differ from country to country. This conditions the type of actions that can be undertaken. For example, South Korea modified its regulations in 2015 due to the MERS crisis, a coronavirus prior to that of 2020. This reform allows competent authorities to access the personal information of each citizen, such as their location and medical reports, in the case of health emergencies (Park et al., 2020). In other regions, however, the legislation is much more restrictive. In the European Union, these applications must comply with the General Data Protection Regulation[18] and the Directive on Privacy and Electronic Communications.[19] These regulations are stricter than those in other territories. Therefore, the same type of measures cannot be taken.

In addition, the crowd may be reluctant to share certain information. According to the study by Alorwu et al. (2020), individuals are more willing to share certain types of personal data than others in crowdsourcing. In particular, they are more likely to share information regarding their religion, racial identity, political opinion, and minor health-related issues, such as a cold, while they are more reluctant to provide information such as their email address, location, last name, and more serious illnesses. These results are surprising given that the latter, with the exception of the health condition, are usually requested in numerous calls that take place on the Internet. The participants in this study argue that this type of information facilitates their identification and that, under anonymity, they are willing to provide information classified as sensitive.

Perhaps, that is where the key to encouraging participation in tracing applications lies: in ensuring that users' identities are not revealed. This should be taken into account when designing applications that monitor the evolution of the pandemic based on the aggregation of data obtained through crowdsourcing. Those responsible for this work must ensure that the privacy of participants is maintained and clearly stated. Otherwise, the crowd may avoid intervening in the activity. In addition, it should be noted that the willingness of individuals to share personal information may have been altered by the pandemic. Some information may be hidden for fear that it will not be viewed well socially, while other information that is normally kept private may be shared for the common good (Nabity-Grover et al., 2020).

In short, achieving participation is of great importance. The success of crowdsourcing is related to the volume of participants it manages to attract. In the case of tracing projects, the greater the number of active users is, the greater the amount of information available for action. However, according to the study by Ferretti et al. (2020), it is not necessary for the entire population to participate. Their results suggest that the epidemic can be contained even if only part of the population is involved. In any case, a sufficient number of users must be attracted.

3.5.5 Duplicated tasks

Crowdsourcing is a very useful tool for collecting data for scientific studies. Thanks to this, part of the process can be streamlined, and more people can be reached (Sheehan, 2018). Studies have shown that crowdsourcing is a reliable technique for this purpose (Strickland and Stoops, 2019). Therefore, it is not surprising that numerous investigations concerning COVID-19 have made use of this tool.

In this context, it may happen that the lines of research of different groups coincide. If both resort to crowdsourcing to obtain the information to be analyzed, two calls are created with the same purpose. If the tasks they propose to the crowd are quite similar, it can be said that there is a duplication in the task. The duplication of contributions is a problem that has been analyzed from an academic point of view. It is a consequence of the dishonest behavior of two or more participants who send the same contribution to obtain a benefit in return. As a consequence, crowdsourcing quality is reduced (Chen et al., 2018).

The duplication of tasks, on the other hand, has not been studied. It is difficult for two calls to coincide. In such a case, a participant must decide whether to participate in both or only in one. In the latter case, the participant must choose one of the them. If there is no reward in return, as is usually the case in these investigations, there is no incentive to participate in both, and an individual can obtain the satisfaction derived from altruism by collaborating in only one. In such a case, both projects would be affected since the crowd willing to participate would be divided into two.

This has happened during the coronavirus crisis. There have been crowdsourcing projects designed to collect similar data within the same health field but managed by different entities. One example is the COVID-19 Sounds App[20] and COVID Voice Detector.[21] These calls aim to develop algorithms to detect the disease through voice. To do this, they need to collect recordings of many volunteers, both healthy and sick. The first belongs to the University of Cambridge (United Kingdom) and the second to Carnegie Mellon University (United States). The tasks they propose to the crowd are very similar. They consist of sending a voice sample: speaking, breathing, and coughing. The crowds they address are almost the same and are global in scale. The COVID-19 Sounds App asks any individual over the age of 16 to participate. The COVID Voice Detector, on the other hand, sets the minimum age for participation at 18. Both indicate that contributions received can be shared with other researchers. However, there is no evidence that they collaborate with each other. It is unlikely that an individual will participate in both. Therefore, it is possible to think that the existence of both acts against the projects since the number of participants each receives would be greater if the other had not been launched. It should be noted that the first results obtained from the COVID-19 Sounds App were published in July 2020 (Brown et al., 2020).

However, if two crowdsourcers discover that they are collecting the same information, they may decide to collaborate. By pooling the contributions they have both received, the volume of data available for research becomes much greater, and both benefit. This has happened with two studies focused on the impact of COVID-19 on chronic liver disease patients: SECURE-Cirrhosis[22] and COVID-Hep.net.[23] The first is managed by a team of doctors from several universities in the United States and involves doctors from America, as well as from China, Japan, Korea, and Mongolia. The second is managed by a group from the University of Oxford (the United Kingdom) and addresses its call to practitioners from the rest of the world, excluding the above territories. Both teams collaborate with each other to achieve the widest possible range and the most reliable results. On their respective websites, they indicate that they work jointly with the other entity. In addition, they warn that you must collaborate with the other researchers if you are not in one of the regions they are in charge of and they add the link to access their site.

Notes

1 www.ushahidi.com
2 www.petabencana.id
3 www.innocentive.com
4 www.covid.postera.ai
5 www.gofundme.com
6 www.foldingathome.org
7 www.innocentive.com
8 www.ennomotive.com
9 www.desafios.enap.gov.br

10 https://covid19.spaceappschallenge.org/
11 www.hackthecrisis.lt
12 www.garage48.org
13 The term "phishing" refers to the deception of users through the Internet. The fraudster, called a phisher, poses as an individual or entity to gain the victim's trust and get the victim to perform certain actions that allow the phisher to steal information.
14 www.cti-league.com
15 www.immuni.italia.it
16 www.stayawaycovid.pt
17 www.coronawarn.app
18 Regulation (EU) 2016/679 of the European Parliament and of the Council of April 27, 2016, on the protection of individuals with regard to the processing of personal data and on the free movement of such data and repealing Directive 95/46/EC *Official Journal of the European Union,* May 4, 2016, N. 119.
19 Directive 2002/58/EC of the European Parliament and of the Council of June 12, 2002, concerning the processing of personal data and the protection of privacy in the electronic communications sector.
20 www.covid-19-sounds.org
21 https://cvd.lti.cmu.edu
22 www.covidcirrhosis.web.unc.edu
23 www.covid-hep.net

Bibliographic references

Acar, O. A. (2019). Motivations and solution appropriateness in crowdsourcing challenges for innovation. *Research Policy, 48*(8), 103716.

Alam, S. L., Sun, R., & Campbell, J. (2020). Helping yourself or others? Motivation dynamics for high-performing volunteers in GLAM crowdsourcing. *Australasian Journal of Information Systems, 24.*

Alorwu, A., van Berkel, N., Goncalves, J., Oppenlaender, J., López, M. B., Seetharaman, M., & Hosio, S. (2020). Crowdsourcing sensitive data using public displays-opportunities, challenges, and considerations. *Personal and Ubiquitous Computing.* https://doi.org/10.1007/s00779-020-01375-6.

Anthony, K. E. (2018). An international crowdsourcing and crisis mapping platform. In A. V. Laskin (Ed.), *Social, mobile, and emerging media around the world: Communication case studies* (pp. 95–107). Lanham, MD: Lexington Books.

Bakici, T. (2020). Comparison of crowdsourcing platforms from social-psychological and motivational perspectives. *International Journal of Information Management, 54,* 102121.

Bieber, J. [@justinbieber]. (2020, May 1). *Help us make the #StuckwithU video: I want to see you guys having fun in quarantine. This is the prom song for everyone who can't go to prom now. Tweet us videos using #stuckwithu or #stuckwithuvideo of you in* [Instagram Video]. Retrieved September 2, 2020, from https://www.instagram.com/p/B_qTChiHfdJ/?utm_source=ig_embed

Blohm, I., Zogaj, S., Bretschneider, U., & Leimeister, J. M. (2018). How to manage crowdsourcing platforms effectively? *California Management Review, 60*(2), 122–149.

Brown, C., Chauhan, J., Grammenos, A., Han, J., Hasthanasombat, A., Spathis, D., . . . Mascolo, C. (2020). Exploring automatic diagnosis of COVID-19 from crowdsourced respiratory sound data. In *Proceedings of the 26th ACM SIGKDD international conference on knowledge discovery & data mining (KDD 2020)* (pp. 1–2). New York: ACM.

Calori, A., & Federici, F. (2020). Coronavirus and beyond: Empowering social self-organization in urban food systems. *Agriculture and Human Values, 14,* 1–2.

Candi, M., Roberts, D. L., Marion, T., & Barczak, G. (2018). Social strategy to gain knowledge for innovation. *British Journal of Management, 29*(4), 731–749.

Cappa, F., Oriani, R., Pinelli, M., & De Massis, A. (2019a). When does crowdsourcing benefit firm stock market performance? *Research Policy, 48*(9), 103825.

Cappa, F., Rosso, F., & Hayes, D. (2019b). Monetary and social rewards for crowdsourcing. *Sustainability, 11*(10), 2834.

Cellini, N., Canale, N., Mioni, G., & Costa, S. (2020). Changes in sleep pattern, sense of time and digital media use during COVID-19 lockdown in Italy. *Journal of Sleep Research,* e13074.

Chason, R. (2020, March 24). Coronavirus leads hospitals, volunteers to crowdsource. *The Washington Post.* Retrieved September 9, 2020, from https://www.washingtonpost.com/local/social-issues/donate-ppe-hospitals-gloves-masks-doctors-nurses/2020/03/23/d781e4cc-6d00-11ea-aa80-c2470c6b2034_story.html

Chen, P. P., Sun, H. L., Fang, Y. L., & Huai, J. P. (2018). Collusion-proof result inference in crowdsourcing. *Journal of Computer Science and Technology, 33*(2), 351–365.

Chen, Q., Min, C., Zhang, W., Wang, G., Ma, X., & Evans, R. (2020). Unpacking the black box: How to promote citizen engagement through government social media during the COVID-19 crisis. *Computers in Human Behavior, 110,* 106380.

Chen, Y. M. (2019). Motivational design in translation crowdsourcing: A gamification approach to Facebook community translation. *Compilation & Translation Review, 12*(1), 141–176.

Christensen, I., & Karlsson, C. (2019). Open innovation and the effects of crowdsourcing in a pharma ecosystem. *Journal of Innovation & Knowledge, 4*(4), 240–247.

Cohen, I. G., Gostin, L. O., & Weitzner, D. J. (2020). Digital smartphone tracking for COVID-19: Public health and civil liberties in tension. *JAMA, 323*(23), 2371–2372.

De', R., Pandey, N., & Pal, A. (2020). Impact of digital surge during Covid-19 pandemic: A viewpoint on research and practice. *International Journal of Information Management, 55,* 102171.

Deng, X. N., & Joshi, K. D. (2016). Why individuals participate in micro-task crowdsourcing work environment: Revealing crowdworkers' perceptions. *Journal of the Association for Information Systems, 17*(10), 711–736.

Directive 2002/58/EC of the European Parliament and the Council, June 12, 2002, concerning the processing of personal data and the protection of privacy in the electronic communications sector.

Droit-Volet, S., Gil, S., Martinelli, N., Andant, N., Clinchamps, M., Parreira, L., . . . Pereira, B. (2020). Time and Covid-19 stress in the lockdown situation: Time free, "Dying" of boredom and sadness. *PloS One, 15*(8), e0236465.

Dwivedi, Y. K., Hughes, D. L., Coombs, C., Constantiou, I., Duan, Y., Edwards, J. S., . . . Raman, R. (2020). Impact of COVID-19 pandemic on information management research and practice: Transforming education, work and life. *International Journal of Information Management, 55,* 102211.

Ebrahim, A. H., & Buheji, M. (2020). A pursuit for a 'holistic social responsibility strategic framework' addressing COVID-19 pandemic needs. *American Journal of Economics*, *10*(5), 293–304.

Ennomotive. (2020). *Respiradores UCI válidos para COVID-19: Desafío Diseño*. Retrieved September 10, 2020, from https://www.ennomotive.com/es/respiradores-uci-covid-19/

Facebook Newsroom [@fbnewsroom]. (2020, March 17). *Joint industry statement from @Facebook, @google, @LinkedIn, @Microsoft, @reddit, @Twitter and @YouTube [Tweet]*. Retrieved September 3, 2020, from https://twitter.com/fbnewsroom/status/123970 3497479614466

Fagherazzi, G., Goetzinger, C., Rashid, M. A., Aguayo, G. A., & Huiart, L. (2020). Digital health strategies to fight COVID-19 worldwide: Challenges, recommendations, and a call for papers. *Journal of Medical Internet Research*, *22*(6), e19284.

Ferretti, L., Wymant, C., Kendall, M., Zhao, L., Nurtay, A., Abeler-Dörner, L., . . . Fraser, C. (2020). Quantifying SARS-CoV-2 transmission suggests epidemic control with digital contact tracing. *Science*, *368*(6491), eabb6936.

Fullana, M. A., Hidalgo-Mazzei, D., Vieta, E., & Radua, J. (2020). Coping behaviors associated with decreased anxiety and depressive symptoms during the COVID-19 pandemic and lockdown. *Journal of Affective Disorders*, *275*, 80–81.

Ghezzi, A., Gabelloni, D., Martini, A., & Natalicchio, A. (2018). Crowdsourcing: A review and suggestions for future research. *International Journal of Management Reviews*, *20*(2), 343–363.

Gooch, D., Kelly, R. M., Stiver, A., van der Linden, J., Petre, M., Richards, M., . . . Walton, C. (2020). The benefits and challenges of using crowdfunding to facilitate community-led projects in the context of digital civics. *International Journal of Human-Computer Studies*, *134*, 33–43.

Google. (2020). *Exposure notifications: Using technology to help public health authorities fight COVID-19*. Google COVID-19 information & resources. Retrieved September 16, 2020, from https://www.google.com/covid19/exposurenotifications/

Grande, A. [@arianagrande]. (2020a, May 7). *Tonight ! #stuckwithu I can't fully articulate ....howwwww happy i am that we waited this long to do this* [Instagram Video]. Retrieved September 2, 2020, from https://www.instagram.com/p/B_5MeJUF1c9/

Grande, A. [@arianagrande]. (2020b, May 8). *Ariana Grande & Justin Bieber - stuck with U* [Video]. Retrieved September 2, 2020, from https://youtu.be/pE49WK-oNjU

Hannewijk, B., Vinella, F. L., Khan, V. J., Lykourentzou, I., Papangelis, K., & Masthoff, J. (2020). Capturing the city's heritage on-the-go: Design requirements for mobile crowdsourced cultural heritage. *Sustainability*, *12*, 2429.

Haroon, O., & Rizvi, S. A. R. (2020). COVID-19: Media coverage and financial markets behavior-A sectoral inquiry. *Journal of Behavioral and Experimental Finance*, *27*, 100343.

Hassan, N. H., & Rahim, F. A. (2017). The rise of crowdsourcing using social media platforms: Security and privacy issues. *Pertanika Journal of Science & Technology*, *25*, 79–88.

Havas, C., Resch, B., Francalanci, C., Pernici, B., Scalia, G., Fernandez-Marquez, J. L., . . . Kirsch, B. (2017). E2mc: Improving emergency management service practice through social media and crowdsourcing analysis in near real time. *Sensors*, *17*(12), 2766.

Hu, F., Bijmolt, T. H., & Huizingh, E. K. (2020). The impact of innovation contest briefs on the quality of solvers and solutions. *Technovation*, 90–91, 102099.

Hunt, A., & Specht, D. (2019). Crowdsourced mapping in crisis zones: Collaboration, organisation and impact. *Journal of International Humanitarian Action*, 4, 1.

Ilmi, Z., Wijaya, A., Kasuma, J., & Darma, D. C. (2020). The crowdsourcing data for innovation. *European Journal of Management Issues*, 28(1–2), 3–12.

InnoCentive. (2020). *COVID-19 challenges*. Retrieved September 3, 2020, from https://www.innocentive.com/covid-19/

INTERPOL. (2020, August). *COVID-19 cybercrime analysis report*. Retrieved September 4, 2020, from https://www.interpol.int/News-and-Events/News/2020/INTERPOL-report-shows-alarming-rate-of-cyberattacks-during-COVID-19

Jacobs, A. (2020, May 11). App shows promise in tracking new coronavirus cases, study finds. *The New York Times*. Retrieved September 9, 2020, from https://www.nytimes.com/2020/05/11/health/coronavirus-symptoms-app.html

Jespersen, K. R. (2018). Crowdsourcing design decisions for optimal integration into the company innovation system. *Decision Support Systems*, 115, 52–63.

Jiang, Z., Huang, Y., & Beil, D. R. (2021). The role of problem specification in crowdsourcing contests for design problems: A theoretical and empirical analysis. *Manufacturing & Service Operations Management*, 23(3), 637–656.

John-Matthews, J. S., Robinson, L., Martin, F., Newton, P. M., & Grant, A. J. (2020). Crowdsourcing: A novel tool to elicit the student voice in the curriculum design process for an undergraduate diagnostic radiography degree programme. *Radiography*, 26, S54–S61.

Kim, E., Fox, S., Moretti, M., Turner, M., Girard, T., & Chan, S. Y. (2019). Motivations and barriers associated with physician volunteerism for an international telemedicine organization. *Frontiers in Public Health*, 7, 224.

Komninos, A. (2019). Pro-social behaviour in crowdsourcing systems: Experiences from a field deployment for beach monitoring. *International Journal of Human-Computer Studies*, 124, 93–115.

Liu, Q., Zheng, Z., Zheng, J., Chen, Q., Liu, G., Chen, S., . . . Zhang, C. J. (2020). Health communication through news media during the early stage of the COVID-19 outbreak in China: Digital topic modeling approach. *Journal of Medical Internet Research*, 22(4), e19118.

Ludwig, T., Kotthaus, C., Reuter, C., Van Dongen, S., & Pipek, V. (2017). Situated crowdsourcing during disasters: Managing the tasks of spontaneous volunteers through public displays. *International Journal of Human-Computer Studies*, 102, 103–121.

Luo, T., Kanhere, S. S., Huang, J., Das, S. K., & Wu, F. (2017). Sustainable incentives for mobile crowdsensing: Auctions, lotteries, and trust and reputation systems. *IEEE Communications Magazine*, 55(3), 68–74.

Mackolil, J., & Mackolil, J. (2020). Addressing psychosocial problems associated with the COVID-19 lockdown. *Asian Journal of Psychiatry*, 51, 102156.

Malhotra, A., Majchrzak, A., Bonfield, W., & Myers, S. (2020). Engaging customer care employees in internal collaborative crowdsourcing: Managing the inherent tensions and associated challenges. *Human Resource Management*, 59(2), 121–134.

Martínez, M. G. (2017). Inspiring crowdsourcing communities to create novel solutions: Competition design and the mediating role of trust. *Technological Forecasting and Social Change*, 117, 296–304.

Menn, J. (2020, March 26). Cybersecurity experts come together to fight coronavirus-related hacking. *Reuters*. Retrieved September 3, 2020, from https://www.reuters.com/article/us-coronavirus-cyber/cybersecurity-experts-come-together-to-fight-coronavirus-related-hacking-idUSKBN21D049

Nabity-Grover, T., Cheung, C. M., & Thatcher, J. B. (2020). Inside out and outside in: How the COVID-19 pandemic affects self-disclosure on social media. *International Journal of Information Management, 55*, 102188.

NASA. (2020a, July 9). *Welcome to NASA@WORK*. Retrieved September 13, 2020, from https://www.nasa.gov/coeci/nasa-at-work

NASA. (2020b, April 1). *NASA taps workforce for innovative ideas for Coronavirus response efforts*. Retrieved September 10, 2020, from https://www.nasa.gov/directorates/spacetech/nasa-taps-workforce-for-innovative-ideas-for-coronavirus-response-efforts

Nevo, D., & Kotlarsky, J. (2020). Crowdsourcing as a strategic IS sourcing phenomenon: Critical review and insights for future research. *Journal of Strategic Information Systems, 29*(4), 101593.

Ni, M. Y., Yang, L., Leung, C. M., Li, N., Yao, X. I., Wang, Y., . . . Liao, Q. (2020). Mental health, risk factors, and social media use during the COVID-19 epidemic and cordon sanitaire among the community and health professionals in Wuhan, China: Cross-sectional survey. *JMIR Mental Health, 7*(5), e19009.

Nor, N. M., Othman, N., & Yusof, S. A. M. (2019). Exploring the decision to volunteer online in health virtual community. *International Journal of Business and Management, 3*(5), 11–18.

Norheim-Hagtun, I., & Meier, P. (2010). Crowdsourcing for crisis mapping in Haiti. *Innovations: Technology, Governance, Globalization, 5*(4), 81–89.

Ogden, R. S. (2020). The passage of time during the UK Covid-19 lockdown. *PloS One, 15*(7), e0235871.

Ogie, R. I., Clarke, R. J., Forehead, H., & Perez, P. (2019). Crowdsourced social media data for disaster management: Lessons from the PetaJakarta. org project. *Computers, Environment and Urban Systems, 73*, 108–117.

Park, S., Choi, G. J., & Ko, H. (2020). Information technology-based tracing strategy in response to COVID-19 in South Korea-privacy controversies. *JAMA, 323*(21), 2129–2130.

Patroni, J., von Briel, F., & Recker, J. (2020). Unpacking the social media–driven innovation capability: How consumer conversations turn into organizational innovations. *Information & Management*, 103267.

Peng, L. (2017). Crisis crowdsourcing and China's civic participation in disaster response: Evidence from earthquake relief. *China Information, 31*(3), 327–348.

Pérez-Escoda, A., Jiménez-Narros, C., Perlado-Lamo-de-Espinosa, M., & Pedrero-Esteban, L. M. (2020). Social networks' engagement during the COVID-19 pandemic in Spain: Health media vs. healthcare professionals. *International Journal of Environmental Research and Public Health, 17*, 5261.

Petri, A. E. (2020, March 31). D.I.Y. Coronavirus solutions are gaining steam. *The New York Times*. Retrieved September 9, 2020, from https://www.nytimes.com/2020/03/31/science/coronavirus-masks-equipment-crowdsource.html

Poblet, M., García-Cuesta, E., & Casanovas, P. (2018). Crowdsourcing roles, methods and tools for data-intensive disaster management. *Information Systems Frontiers, 20*(6), 1363–1379.

Pyle, A. S., Morgoch, M. L., & Boatwright, B. C. (2019). SnowedOut Atlanta: Examining digital emergence on facebook during a crisis. *Journal of Contingencies and Crisis Management, 27*(4), 414–422.

Ratner, L., Martin-Blais, R., Warrell, C., & Narla, N. P. (2020). Reflections on resilience during the COVID-19 pandemic: Six lessons from working in resource-denied settings. *The American Journal of Tropical Medicine and Hygiene, 102*(6), 1178–1180.

Regulation (EU) 2016/679 of the European Parliament and of the Council of April 27, 2016 on the protection of individuals with regard to the processing of personal data and on the free movement of such data and repealing Directive 95/46/EC *Official Journal of the European Union*, May 4, 2016, N. 119.

Riccardi, M. T. (2016). The power of crowdsourcing in disaster response operations. *International Journal of Disaster Risk Reduction, 20*, 123–128.

Rodríguez-Rey, R., Garrido-Hernansaiz, H., & Collado, S. (2020). Psychological impact and associated factors during the initial stage of the Coronavirus (COVID-19) pandemic among the general population in Spain. *Frontiers in Psychology, 11*, 1540.

Sheehan, K. B. (2018). Crowdsourcing research: Data collection with Amazon's mechanical turk. *Communication Monographs, 85*(1), 140–156.

Sheehan, K. B., & Pittman, M. (2019). Straight from the source? Media framing of creative crowd labor and resultant ethical concerns. *Journal of Business Ethics, 154*(2), 575–585.

Sinha, M., Pande, B., & Sinha, R. (2020). Impact of COVID-19 lockdown on sleep-wake schedule and associated lifestyle related behavior: A national survey. *Journal of Public Health Research, 9*(3).

Song, P., & Karako, T. (2020). Scientific solidarity in the face of the COVID-19 pandemic: Researchers, publishers, and medical associations. *Global Health & Medicine, 2*(2), 56–59.

Standing, S., & Standing, C. (2018). The ethical use of crowdsourcing. *Business Ethics: A European Review, 27*(1), 72–80.

Strickland, J. C., & Stoops, W. W. (2019). The use of crowdsourcing in addiction science research: Amazon mechanical turk. *Experimental and Clinical Psychopharmacology, 27*(1), 1–18.

Sun, K., Chen, J., & Viboud, C. (2020). Early epidemiological analysis of the coronavirus disease 2019 outbreak based on crowdsourced data: A population-level observational study. *The Lancet Digital Health, 2*(4), e201–e208.

Thuan, N. H., Antunes, P., & Johnstone, D. (2016). Factors influencing the decision to crowdsource: A systematic literature review. *Information Systems Frontiers, 18*(1), 47–68.

Thuan, N. H., Antunes, P., & Johnstone, D. (2017). A process model for establishing business process crowdsourcing. *Australasian Journal of Information Systems, 21*, 1–21.

Tucker, J. D., Pan, S. W., Mathews, A., Stein, G., Bayus, B., & Rennie, S. (2018). Ethical concerns of and risk mitigation strategies for crowdsourcing contests and innovation challenges: Scoping review. *Journal of Medical Internet Research, 20*(3), e75.

UN-Habitat. (2020, June 12). *COVID-19 campaign survey*. Retrieved September 2, 2020, from https://storymaps.arcgis.com/collections/271338c7ea284def89e4fb066c89529b?item=1.

University of Chicago. (2020). *UChicago crowdsourcing COVID-19 history*. Retrieved September 6, 2020, from https://www.uchicago.hk/alumni/uchicago-crowd-sourcing-of-history-covid-19/

Ushahidi. (n.d.). *Crisis preparedness platform*. Retrieved August 31, 2020, from https://www.ushahidi.com/case-studies/crisis-preparedness-platform

Usher, A. D. (2020). WHO launches crowdfund for COVID-19 response. *The Lancet, 395*(10229), 1024.

Wang, X., Goh, D. H. L., & Lim, E. P. (2020). Understanding continuance intention toward crowdsourcing games: A longitudinal investigation. *International Journal of Human-Computer Interaction, 36*(12), 1168–1177.

Wehn, U., & Almomani, A. (2019). Incentives and barriers for participation in community-based environmental monitoring and information systems: A critical analysis and integration of the literature. *Environmental Science & Policy, 101*, 341–357.

Weil, T., & Murugesan, S. (2020). IT risk and resilience-cybersecurity response to COVID-19. *IEEE Computer Architecture Letters, 22*(3), 4–10.

World Health Organization. (2020a, January 5). *Emergency preparedness and response: Pneumonia of unknown cause - China*. Retrieved September 10, 2020, from https://www.who.int/csr/don/05-january-2020-pneumonia-of-unkown-cause-china/es/

World Health Organization. (2020b, January 10). *International travel and health: WHO advice on international travel and trade in relation to the outbreak of pneumonia caused by a new coronavirus in China*. Retrieved September 10, 2020, from https://www.who.int/ith/2020-0901_outbreak_of_Pneumonia_caused_by_a_new_coronavirus_in_C/es/

World Health Organization. (2020c, June 29). *Chronology of WHO's response to VIDOC-19*. Retrieved September 10, 2020, from https://www.who.int/es/news-room/detail/29-06-2020-covidtimeline

World Health Organization. (2020d, January 30). *Statement by WHO director-general on the meeting of the international health regulations emergency committee on the new Coronavirus (2019-nCoV)*. Retrieved September 10, 2020, from https://www.who.int/es/dg/speeches/detail/who-director-general-s-statement-on-ihr-emergency-committee-on-novel-coronavirus-(2019-ncov).

World Health Organization. (2020e, March 11). Opening address by the director-general of WHO at the press conference on COVID-19 held on 11 March 2020. Retrieved September 10, 2020, from https://www.who.int/es/dg/speeches/detail/who-director-general-s-opening-remarks-at-the-media-briefing-on-covid-19-11-march-2020

World Health Organization. (2020f). *Questions and answers on contact tracing in the context of COVID-19*. Retrieved September 10, 2020, from https://www.who.int/es/news-room/q-a-detail/q-a-contact-tracing-for-covid-19

Yang, K. (2019). Research on factors affecting solvers' participation time in online crowdsourcing contests. *Future Internet, 11*(8), 176.

Yardley, E., Lynes, A. G. T., Wilson, D., & Kelly, E. (2018). What's the deal with "web-sleuthing"? News media representations of amateur detectives in networked spaces. *Crime Media Culture, 14*(1), 81–109.

Yaseen, S. G., & Al Omoush, K. S. (2020). Mobile crowdsourcing technology acceptance and engagement in crisis management: The case of Syrian refugees. *International Journal of Technology and Human Interaction (IJTHI), 16*(3), 1–23.

4 Crowdsourcing applications during the COVID-19 crisis

4.1 Social area

4.1.1 Applications

One of the possible applications of crowdsourcing is social innovation. For example, collective efforts can be directed at combating inequalities and improving the living conditions of the less advantaged members of a population (Fuger et al., 2017). To mitigate the effects of the pandemic in this area, social resilience can be promoted through citizen cohesion and solidarity. This can be achieved by building a collective capacity to deal with the consequences of confinement. Such efforts also encourage authorities to give visibility to projects that pursue the welfare of the community and to give recognition to the roles that they play during such periods (Elcheroth & Drury, 2020).

In this context, crowdsourcing projects have mainly been created to help the most vulnerable residents of neighborhoods. For example, campaigns have been developed to solicit donations for food banks and soup kitchens, and low-risk populations have been encouraged to help with daily activities such as going to the pharmacy or the supermarket for those belonging to high-risk groups who should not be exposed to the virus, such as the elderly and chronically ill populations (Misra, 2020).

This is often referred to as spatial crowdsourcing, in which tasks must be carried out in a specific location (Liu et al., 2018). Therefore, platforms often use maps that indicate where help is required. The following is a case study in this category in which Ushahidi's technology is used to inform users about the places where collaboration is requested. As previously mentioned, this is a fairly recurrent crowdsourcing platform in crisis management.

DOI: 10.4324/9781003290872-4

4.1.2 Case study: slow the curve

Frena La Curva[1] is a project initiated by the Aragon Open Government Lab (LAAAB), a service of the Government of Aragon (Spain), in March 2020. Its objective is to "accelerate, make visible and multiply citizen projects that help fight the situation caused by COVID-19" (LAAAB, 2020). To this end, their members teamed up with volunteers as entrepreneurs or activists to create the Frena La Curva platform, which is a website that collects and displays these calls. The platform has been a success since its launch; in 48 hours, more than 900 users registered (LAAAB, 2020). The platform consists of several activities. The most important one is the Frena La Curva map. This is a collaborative map that indicates the location of offers and requests for help. This project also has a forum that allows users to dialogue with each other and contribute resources and advice. In addition, platform members have created events and calls to develop new ideas, such as the Frena La Curva Festival, Common Challenges, and the Citizens' Labs. These ideas pursue open innovation and the exchange of ideas.

The project has been replicated in 22 countries, mainly in Latin America. This case study focuses on the Frena La Curva map of Spain. It should be noted that on June 22, 2020, Frena La Curva Spain provided its last update on its Twitter profile. They announced the arrival of the new normal and said goodbye to their followers (Frena La Curva, 2020b). Despite the fact that no deadline was set for participation, the evolution of the pandemic means that the activity is no longer necessary.

4.1.2.1 Crowdsourcing elements

CROWDSOURCER

The idea for Frena La Curva came from the Aragon Open Government Lab during the days prior to home confinement in Spain. Other agents, such as companies, social organizations, citizens' associations, and other public innovation laboratories such as the one in Aragon, soon joined in. Two of the first to join were the companies of Impact Hub, which defines itself as "the largest global network of entrepreneurial communities with impact, present in 55 countries around the world" (Impact Hub, n.d.), and Las Naves, which is a public entity that depends on the city council of Valencia (Spain) and promotes social innovation through participation. In the first 24 hours, agents from almost all areas of Spain joined in. To manage the project, these agents created a coordination group.

PLATFORM

First, the website of Frena La Curva was created to help collect all the citizen projects that were being organized. Days later, the map was developed. The map shows both offers of help and the needs of the population. It uses Ushahidi technology. The information is visualized using the OpenStreetMap program. The web version of the map can be accessed from either a computer or an application accessed through a mobile device. This platform was created specifically for this activity but utilizes existing resources. Furthermore, since it is based on free software tools, it can be easily and cheaply replicated in other countries (Kaleidos, 2020a, 2020b).

TASKS

The Frena La Curva map acts as a link between aid requesters and volunteers. That is, it represents an open platform where many people ask a multitude of collaborators to carry out some task for them. This need can be one of their own or an act of mediation for someone else in need. In the first case, the individual who requires help provides information about their need through the Frena La Curva questionnaire. In the second case, a third-party person provides information about the need of another person. On the other hand, users can show their offers of help and establish which tasks they are willing to carry out for others. In addition, it is possible to indicate the existence of available public services whose schedules have been modified, such as social centers that offer food or stores that sell essential items, among others.

Some examples of needs and offerings are buying food or medicine, taking out the garbage, preparing food, or providing accompaniment via the telephone. All of these are reflected on the map by the presence of pins. The pin color varies depending on who creates it. Those who request help with a need are red or, if the help was requested by a third-party member, orange. Offers of help have a green color. Finally, public services are differentiated by the color blue. It should be noted that the pins can be removed at any time.

PARTICIPANTS

Participation is open to everyone, including public institutions, companies, nonprofit organizations, citizens' associations, and individuals. Anyone can collaborate on this platform. The only requirement is to have a device with an Internet connection to access the map. Although this requirement is common to all projects, crowdsourcing is based on the use of new technologies.

4.1.2.2 Favorable conditions

MOTIVATED PARTICIPANTS

The main motivation to participate is altruism. Some people are suffering more than others from the effects of the pandemic, especially vulnerable populations who are not able to care for themselves or for whom it is more dangerous to be exposed to the virus. Frena La Curva calls for voluntary action to improve the conditions of these neighborhood populations. It does not provide anything in return for participation, only the satisfaction of having helped someone else.

It should be noted that Frena La Curva has a complementary forum through which participants can share information and interests as appropriate during the pandemic. Its purpose is to create a virtual community for knowledge sharing through conversations and discussions about projects that combat the effects of the coronavirus, such as other neighborhood support networks, websites, and resources to facilitate one's adaptation to the new conditions arising from the pandemic. Participants may ask questions, and others may provide comments or another questions in regard to these queries. Recognition in the form of a badge is given to the most active users. In this way, these users gain a reputation in the community. This serves as an incentive. In addition, the forum allows contact with other people. Therefore, this tool helps to meet the need of socializing with other individuals during the period of confinement.

TIME TO PARTICIPATE

Before performing a task, a volunteer must register his or her offer or seek out the needs of others. This task requires little time to complete, as only a few details need to be provided. However, the time that must be dedicated to carrying out this task varies and depends on different factors. For example, aid requesters have different needs. It does not take the same amount of time to take out the garbage as it does to go to a store and make a purchase. In addition, the volunteer has to travel to the home of the individual who needs help, and the travel time depends on the distance. In any case, such travel is not a short task. Therefore, Frena La Curva benefits from the increased amount of free time derived from confinement. In everyday life before the pandemic, some people may have been interested in working with a neighborhood aid organization but did not have the time to do so. Teleworking and the impossibility of carrying out leisure activities outside the home have allowed these individuals to take part in such activities.

EASE OF DISSEMINATION

Frena La Curva has profiles on the social network platforms of Twitter and Facebook. From its website, the platform encourages users to share their content on both of them. In this way, users help increase the possibility that a greater percentage of the population knows about the project and decides to participate. In addition, different Spanish media have reported on this. These include written media such as the El País and La Razón newspapers, television channels such as La Sexta and radio channels such as Cadena Cope (Frena La Curva, 2020c). Finally, the Frena La Curva has a channel in the Telegram app that is of great help with regard to spreading and recreating this project in other countries.

CROWDSOURCER'S EXPERIENCE

The organizers have different profiles that range from companies to citizen associations. Many of them have experience in crowdsourcing and open innovation. Aragon Open Government Lab, the initiator institution, is a tool for democratic innovation that promotes citizen participation in the design of public policies. Las Naves has innovation networks and collaborative spaces that actively involve citizens in the development of new projects. The company Impact Hub connects its members and promotes entrepreneurship and innovation programs. The company Kaleidos has a similar mission but is focused on the technological level.

OPEN RESOURCES

Open resources do not bring any benefit to this project given the characteristics of its task.

NO ECONOMIC BENEFIT FOR THE CROWDSOURCER

Frena La Curva is not for profit. It has been created thanks to the collaboration of many entities that aim to give visibility to citizens' projects. The organizers act in a disinterested way and do not receive remuneration for their work.

4.1.2.3 *Barriers*

NO TIME FOR PLANNING

The design process took place in two phases, which were divided into several steps. Time was pressing, as the population needed to be helped as soon as possible. For this reason, the duration of each of the steps was very short. These steps are explained as follows (Frena La Curva, 2020a):

- Phase 1: Urgent
  - Step 0. Partnerships to create a community: over the course of one or two days, a community of volunteers based on thought and action was created in a network.
  - Step 1. Forum to organize the projects: it took between three and five days to develop a forum to collect all the calls that were taking place.
  - Step 2. Creating impact: Two to four days were spent thinking about how to create direct impact. The members started talking about Citizen Labs and the possibility of using a map.
  - Step 3. Citizens' Labs: In a span of five days, several labs launched calls to promote projects and managed to attract 200 participants. Their aim was to facilitate the initial development of new of them.
  - Step 4. Frena La Curva map: Within two days, the idea of developing a map to connect requests and offers of citizen help using Ushahidi's technology was taken up again. The map was scheduled to be launched on March 20, 2020.

- Phase 2: Important
  - Step 5. Consolidation: work continues to include more projects.
  - Step 6. Growth: Agreements are sought with organizations and associations to increase the impact of Frena La Curva. The call for common challenges is also managed.

The duration of each of the steps of the first phase, labeled "urgent," was equal to or less than five days. The planning of the project was carried out very quickly. Thanks to this, the Frena La Curva map was launched a few days after the start of the movement restrictions in Spain. In this way, it was possible to attend to the requests derived from the confinement almost from the beginning.

DIGITAL DIVIDE

The organizers of Frena La Curva were aware of the problem caused by the digital divide. It based on citizen collaboration can be very useful for vulnerable people, since they are the ones who need these services the most. For this reason, the organizers have added a third option to the function of asking and requesting help, that is, pointing out a need through an intermediary. In this way, one person can give visibility to the request of another who does not have the resources or knowledge to access Frena La Curva.

Moreover, organizers encourage their users to be proactive and to determine if any of their neighbors need this service. They place special emphasis on the elderly population. To this end, they propose that volunteers ask other residents in their building (taking extreme precautions to avoid direct contact) or post an information sign at the building's portal. In this way, volunteers can act as intermediaries.

CYBERATTACKS

There is no record of any cyberattack on Frena La Curva. However, it should be noted that the participants provide very little data, which are not sufficient to identify them. Therefore, the associated risk is low.

SENSITIVE DATA

To create a need or an offer on the Frena La Curva map, they must add location and contact information. The platform makes a series of recommendations to encourage the privacy of its users. Regarding the location, the platform advises giving an approximate address. For example, users are encouraged to share the street on which they live, but not their full address. The platform also points out that if a volunteer provides information that is too detailed, the moderators will delete it. With regard to contact information, the platform suggests giving an email address instead of a phone number, as this is a less invasive means of contact. The moderators also point out that by registering a need or an offer, the user gives his or her consent for the data that he or she has provided to be published publicly on the platform.

DUPLICATED TASKS

There are other crowdsourcing calls with the same purpose as this one, that is, to create a neighborhood support network to soften the effects of the pandemic on the most vulnerable populations. However, the presence of multiple projects can work against the applicants; that is, there may be volunteers in your area who use other platforms to offer their help. In such a case, there is no connection between the parties, and if there is no partner in the area, the need remains unmet. Even so, Frena La Curva aims to give visibility to all existing projects, including those that request the same kind of tasks. It encourages its users to share these calls through its forum. In this way, the impediment of the simultaneous existence of more than one call for the same task can be mitigated.

4.2 Health area

4.2.1 Applications

Many projects related to the health field have been created in this context, such as calls for the manufacture of masks by volunteers or contests that challenge the crowd to design more efficient medical devices. One of the most important applications during this period calls for research on the new virus. One of the advantages of crowdsourcing over traditional methods is the reduction of the time needed to perform a certain task (Hosseini et al., 2019). Speed in identifying problems and finding solutions is paramount in a crisis. The effects of the new coronavirus were unknown at the beginning of the pandemic, and health investigations require long periods of time to be carried out. However, the option of carrying out such investigations has largely not been available under the circumstances of the pandemic.

Therefore, crowdsourcing represents a powerful tool to learn more about the disease. On the one hand, information can be collected and analyzed more quickly, speeding up both phases of such studies (Leung & Leung, 2020). Crowdsourcing also favors the quality of innovations and improves the learning capacity and access to knowledge (Ahn et al., 2019). This approach is key at times of crises. Solutions must not only be found quickly but also be effective. Crowdsourcing has been implemented for different purposes in this context.

For example, it has been used to define what impact the disease has on patients with other preexisting illnesses. For this purpose, international registries have been created that allow the medical community to report on what symptoms these patients are presenting. The aim is to identify the evolution, possible complications, and outcomes related to such patients. There are projects aimed at investigating how COVID-19 affects those suffering from inflammatory bowel disease,[2] celiac disease,[3] or rheumatic diseases,[4] among others. Most of them are organized by universities in the United States and have collaborators who promote their dissemination in other countries.

Although these studies based on international registries allow preliminary results to be obtained very quickly, they also have limitations. Some of these limitations consist of the absence of a control group, possible duplicated records, or the selective inclusion of cases. Thus, these collaborative projects are not a substitute for rigorous scientific research (Freeman et al., 2020; Robinson & Yadany, 2020).

4.2.2 Case study: COVID Symptom Study app

The COVID Symptom Study app[5] is a crowdsourcing-based application that collects daily information about its users' symptoms. Its download is free and voluntary. The app was created in March 2020 to collect data in the United Kingdom and has been exported to the United States and Sweden. To participate in the study app, you do not need to have a positive diagnosis or a suspicion of suffering from the disease. The data collected are used to investigate the symptoms and the speed of spread, as well as to identify areas at high risk of contagion.

This research is one of the most important applications for symptom monitoring in the population. Numerous findings have emerged from this crowdsourcing research and have been published in major scientific journals. So great is the success of this app that in August 2020, it was announced that the Department of Health and Social Welfare of England is giving the organizers a grant of two million pounds to continue the study during the winter (ZOE, 2020f).

This application should not be confused with the NHS Test and Trace app,[6] which is the official contact tracing application of the UK's National Health Service (NHS). The NHS app uses Bluetooth technology from the users' cell phones and the API developed by Google and Apple. The COVID Symptom Study app, on the other hand, does not trace the contacts of an individual with a positive diagnosis. It only collects data about symptoms that its users voluntarily submit.

4.2.2.1 Crowdsourcing elements

CROWDSOURCER

The app was organized by ZOE, a health science company, in collaboration with King's College London, which is in charge of the research. Although it is independent of government agencies, the app is endorsed by the governments and national health services of Wales and Scotland. The application provides daily data updates on infections, risk areas, and prevalence rates to the governments of the United Kingdom, Wales, and Scotland. In other words, the app was developed by a private company, but it collaborates with public institutions. On the other hand, the US replica was created by ZOE in collaboration with King's College in London, Massachusetts General Hospital, Harvard School of Public Health, and Stanford University Medical School.

PLATFORM

The platform was developed by ZOE. It is a mobile application designed specifically for this purpose. Therefore, it is a proprietary platform. You can only participate through mobile devices, since these devices are the only ones that allow the download of the app; the developers have not launched a web version. The app is available in Apple Store and Google Play. That is, the organizers have adapted it to both major operating systems. In addition, it is intended that the app's users access it periodically. Therefore, they added a feature that sends reminders to them.

TASK

The task is to fill out a questionnaire about one's health status. This is a simple task that requires little time to complete. This is one of the main characteristics of the app. Therefore, the COVID Symptom Study tries to attract population involvement by stating that they can help in the fight against coronavirus by spending just one minute a day on the application. In addition, any individuals can participate since the app does not require specific knowledge or skills to be executed.

PARTICIPANTS

This project aims to involve millions of people (Spector & Chan, 2020). In September 2020, the application was available in the United Kingdom, the United States, and Sweden. Therefore, participation can only take place if you are a resident of one of these countries. In addition, you must have a mobile device to download the app. There are no further restrictions. Anyone can participate regardless of their coronavirus diagnosis. All contributions are valid for analyzing the effects and evolution of the pandemic.

4.2.2.2 Favorable conditions

MOTIVATED PARTICIPANTS

The COVID Symptom Study does not explicitly offer any incentives. The participants are not remunerated for completing the questionnaire nor does the app have any mechanisms related to the reputation of its users, since the update task is performed on the basis of anonymity. Therefore, it can be stated that the main motivation of the participants is altruism. The users collaborate to help scientific research and accelerate the results of studies about coronavirus. In this way, they act for the common good. Research is carried out to learn more about the disease that causes coronavirus. The more that is known, the sooner the crisis will be over.

It should be noted that the total number of users of the application is displayed on the home page of the website. In mid-September, the number of users was over four million. This can motivate other individuals to participate through social influence, that is, through the effect that the actions of others have on the individual. Additionally, the app requires recurrent participation, specifically, on a daily basis. To encourage this involvement, the COVID Symptom Study app sends reminders to its users.

TIME TO PARTICIPATE

One of the favorable conditions for crowdsourcing during this period is the increase in the population's free time as a result of home confinement. However, this free time can be employed in the pursuit other activities instead of participating in the study app. In any case, the COVID Symptom Study requires a very short participation time. In particular, both the website and the application indicate that only one minute a day should be spent on the cause. This is the time needed to answer the app's questionnaire about the user's symptoms. Therefore, any individual can participate regardless of the conditions that surround them. Those who telework, care for others, or have many occupations can dedicate one minute a day to collaborate with the research about the new coronavirus disease.

EASE OF DISSEMINATION

This application has managed to attract a large number of users; more importantly, it did so during the first days after its launch. In just 36 hours, there were more than a million downloads (ZOE, 2020a). This activity made it the most downloaded application from the Google Play Store in the health category (Volpicelli, 2020). In this way, the crowd itself has helped to spread the app. Being at the top of that list gives it visibility, which can help more individuals access it. Additionally, Mark Drakeford, the Welsh Prime Minister, urged citizens to download the application (ZOE, 2020b). Numerous media outlets have echoed this call, including the New York Times (Jacobs, 2020), the BBC (Agerholm, 2020), and the Guardian (Davis, 2020).

On the other hand, the ZOE company has organized several web seminars to publicize the application and the results they have been obtaining thanks to it (ZOE, 2020c). These web seminars were publicized through social network platforms such as Facebook (ZOE, 2020d). In addition, the recordings of these seminars have been published on YouTube so that anyone can access them later. Through this strategy, the call for help is brought even closer to the population. The progress being made in regard to the research on coronavirus is due to the small contributions of the crowd made through the application. Raising awareness of the importance of their collaboration can encourage them to continue to participate and for others to decide to start participating.

CROWDSOURCER'S EXPERIENCE

ZOE is a technology company that was born from the union of Tim Spector, the researcher who directs the COVID Symptom Study; two experts in artificial intelligence and consumer applications; and researchers from major universities in the United Kingdom and the United States. The company offers nutritional advice in a digital way. In addition, it uses the data it collects to carry out studies in this field, whose results have been published in major journals such as *Nature Medicine* (ZOE, 2020e). In other words, the company has experience with crowdsourcing as it applies to research. Tim Spector adapted this model to create the COVID Symptom Study, which, instead of focusing on the nutritional field, focuses on the effects of the new coronavirus.

OPEN RESOURCES

Open resources are not relevant to executing this task since it is simple and no knowledge is needed to perform it. However, it is worth noting that this project has produced numerous findings that have been published in prestigious scientific journals and are part of the resources referred to in regard to this app having a favorable factor for other crowd-sourcing activities.

The COVID Symptom Study app claims to derive no economic benefit from this project. It warns that the data can be shared with other entities, but not for profit. In other words, the app does not commercialize the information of its users. However, the crowdsourcer does achieve a direct benefit, that is, making discoveries regarding the coronavirus and having them published brings about work recognition and an increased reputation within the scientific community.

4.2.2.3 Barriers

NO TIME FOR PLANNING

Tim Spector, the director of this project, also leads TwinsUK research, one of the most important twin studies in the world (TwinsUK, 2020a). At the beginning of the pandemic, his intention was to analyze the effects of the coronavirus on twins as part of this study. To this end, ZOE was commissioned to develop an application in which TwinsUK participants could report their symptoms (TwinsUK, 2020b). The ZOE team thought it might be useful to allow the participation of any individual, not just the twins in the study. They worked with great urgency, and four days later, on March 24, 2020, the COVID Symptom Study app was launched in the United Kingdom (Volpicelli, 2020). The emergency situation caused the app to be created in a very short time. Its developers managed to reduce the planning and design time, thereby allowing its launch to take place just a few days after it was conceived.

DIGITAL DIVIDE

Given its purpose, it was advisable to create some strategy to facilitate the participation of all individuals. To properly study the effects of the virus, a representative group of the population must be examined. However, there are groups within the population that do not have a smartphone and therefore cannot download the application. In addition, there are others who, although they do have a smartphone, do not have suffi-cient skills to download the app. In this situation, no analyzable data are obtained from these subpopulations.

The COVID Symptom Study allows users to create several profiles within it and thus report the symptoms of more than one person through a single device. It encourages the recording of the evolution of other individuals, for example, a user's family members. In addition, the app indicates that these individuals must be asked for their consent to do so. In addition, the platform warns that users must download the latest version of the application to enter more than one profile. This suggests that the previous versions of the app did not have this functionality. This is, this strategy of inclusion emerged during the process of improving the project.

Even so, users can only participate through the application; the website does not have that functionality. Therefore, you can only collaborate if you have a mobile device on which to download the app.

CYBERATTACKS

While there has been an increase in the number of cyberattacks during the pandemic, there is no reference to any of them being directed at this project. Additionally, the study website states that precautions have been taken to prevent such attacks and to protect participants' data, although that risk cannot be entirely eliminated.

SENSITIVE DATA

The contributions required include the provision of sensitive data, such as one's health status. The crowdsourcers state that they only request the information necessary to carry out the study and that they have tried to minimize the information needed. They give as an example data referring to age. Participants must indicate their year of birth. However, to reduce the data that could allow their identification, the COVID Symptom Study does not ask participants to provide their day of birth.

The app is also governed by the European Union's General Data Protection Regulations, even though the data, after processing them to make them anonymous, are shared with institutions in the United States. In this territory, the regulations are less restrictive. This is stated on the platform's website. The organizers also state that participants have agreed to this sharing through the consent they have given through the application. It should be noted that the platform gives its users the possibility to revoke this consent at any time.

DUPLICATED TASKS

Research into the effects of the coronavirus on the population is one of the main measures being undertaken to curb the pandemic. Crowdsourcing is a very useful tool for this purpose given the mobility restrictions that existed during the beginning of this pandemic period. Therefore, it is not strange that multiple projects have been created that request a very similar task from the population. Since there are other studies focusing on coronavirus symptoms, the COVID Symptom Study states that it is collaborating with other researchers from several countries and coordinating their efforts to speed up the research.

4.3 Educational area

4.3.1 Applications

The education sector has been greatly impacted by the pandemic. Most schools closed their doors during the first few months of the pandemic to curb the effects of the coronavirus. As a result, more than 1.5 billion students have been affected (UNESCO, 2020). Education has had to be transferred to the digital world in order to continue. Thus, COVID-19 has represented an opportunity to accelerate the digital transformation of this sector. However, this transformation requires that both teachers and students have certain resources, such as electronic devices and Internet access (Mulenga & Marbán, 2020). Not all homes have a device available for the students who live there to access virtual classes.

Crowdsourcing has been used to close this gap. For example, the local administration of the municipality Câmara de Lobos (Portugal) made call to its inhabitants through Facebook for the donation of computers in April 2020. The aim was to distribute these computers among disadvantaged families so that all local students could receive an online education (Covid19People, 2020). Another similar project is Take My Laptop, a campaign to collect computers and tablets to give them to students with fewer resources; it was launched in the same month (April 2020) by the Institute of Economic Studies of Alicante (Spain) (Instituto de Estudios Económicos Provincia de Alicante, 2020).

However, those who attend institutions with financial resources or those who are immersed in the digital transformation process are more likely to continue learning. These centers have the capacity to adapt to the new reality and to provide education remotely. On the other hand, students who attend centers with fewer financial resources or more traditional resources are at a disadvantage. Their institutions must make a great effort to adapt to the digital world, and it is likely that, if they do so, the product will be a lower quality of teaching. Therefore, making free content available to any student anywhere in the world is a way to facilitate learning. This can be done through crowdsourcing. This tool can also be used to recruit volunteers to help these students in a selfless way, as seen in the case below.

4.3.2 Case study: Coronavirus Tutoring Project

The Coronavirus Tutoring Project (CTI)[7] was created at the end of March 2020 after the closure of educational centers in the United Kingdom. It aims to provide free tutoring to low-income students who need it during the home confinement. To this end, the developers are appealing for crowdsourcing by focusing on university students willing to do so altruistically. The tutorials take place through digital platforms, thereby respecting the movement restrictions established by the authorities.

4.3.2.1 Crowdsourcing elements

CROWDSOURCER

CTI was born from the union of three students from the University of Oxford and the Project Access team.[8] Project Access is a nonprofit project that helps students from less privileged backgrounds during the application process at prestigious universities. They employ their community of volunteers who are responsible, through individual tutoring, for guiding the applicants.

CTI has been developed to reduce the disparity between students whose families can afford to pay for a private teacher and those who cannot. The closure of schools to prevent the spread of coronavirus has forced the move to digital education. Adapting to this new environment can be complex for students. This is especially true for those who cannot afford to hire outside help.

PLATFORM

The CTI takes place through a set of platforms. On the one hand, it has its own website where it provides information about the project and through which an application to participate can be sent. To do so, the platform relies on a Google Form. In addition, CTI has the support of Bramble[9] and Adapt.[10] Bramble is a digital platform designed to carry out digital tutoring. It is a paid service. Those teachers and organizations who want to use it must pay a fee in return. However, it is free for volunteers, who use it to contact students. On the other hand, Adapt is an application that acts as a planner. It is specially designed for students. It allows you to record class schedules and homework assignments. In addition, it graphically shows the percentage of the activities that has been completed during the day, thereby motivating its users. Unlike Bramble, Adapt is free.

TASK

The task consists of providing individual tutoring to students who request help. This is done through digital platforms, mainly Bramble. The organization of CTI puts both parties in contact, depending on their needs. In addition, the task is carried out in an altruistic way; the tutors do not receive compensation for their work. It should be noted that CTI has created two other complementary projects. First, CTI has placed crowd-funding campaign on its website to obtain funds to finance the main project. Initially, the organizers used the savings of one of their three founders. However, this amount did not turn out to be enough. Therefore, they subsequently devised a call for funding (Robertson, 2020). It can be decided by a user whether his or her donation is made anonymously or not. Thus, anyone can participate. It is not necessary to be a tutor. In fact, the more individuals who donate, the more successful the crowdfunding campaign will be. Second, CTI has a resource bank, and tutors can send in material to help enrich it. This work is voluntary and is done through a Google Form designed specifically for this purpose by the organizers.

PARTICIPANTS

The call for participants is addressed to a specific group of individuals. The first step in becoming a tutor is to send an application through a Google questionnaire available on the CTI website. In addition, only university students can participate. To verify this requirement, individuals must provide their email address from the university where they are studying on the application form. In other words, participation is restricted to a sector of the population. In addition, if a candidate is chosen, he or she must pass a course before tutoring can take place. During the first week, the platform received 3,000 requests from university students to collaborate in the project; and the participants have provided more than 20,000 hours of tutoring. After the assignment of students, the volunteers carry out their work individually. They offer their own classes independently. That is, the participants do not compete or collaborate with each other.

4.3.2.2 *Favorable conditions*

MOTIVATED PARTICIPANTS

First, CTI posts photos of some of the volunteers on Twitter, naming them the "tutors of the day." This gives recognition to their work and visibility to their actions. In addition, the platform adds testimonies given by the participants, who point out different motivations for collaborating with CTI. These motivations include spending time on something worthwhile, helping those in need, and learning. They also say that the experience is fun and that they enjoy doing it (CTI, 2020a, 2020b, 2020c). In other words, there are several categories of incentives that encourage participation, and each participant has his or her own reasons for doing so.

TIME TO PARTICIPATE

This task requires much dedication. Considerable time must be invested in tutoring. In addition, participation must be done on a recurring basis. CTI benefits directly from the increased free time during this period. University students, although they have to attend their own virtual classes, study, and work, currently do not spend a part of their day engaging in leisure time outside of the home. However, since this is a very demanding task, volunteers can notify the platform at any time of their desire to reduce the number of hours if they become too busy.

EASE OF DISSEMINATION

The organizers, three students from the University of Oxford, spread the project among their peers. Students from this university represent the highest percentage among the CTI volunteers, followed by those from the University of Cambridge. Such was their initial success that they managed to attract more tutors than students who needed online classes (Robertson, 2020). Therefore, the organizers had to devise a strategy to raise awareness of the project among the students in need. To do so, they used social networks such as Twitter. Through this platform, they asked parents and teachers to provide information about it to students who need this service (CTI, 2020d). This information is intended to be disseminated through informal networks of contacts, that is, through calls and messages between individuals who know about the existence of students who are in this situation.

CROWDSOURCER'S EXPERIENCE

Project Access, one of the organizers, has previous experience with crowdsourcing. Project Access is an entity created in 2016 to help students from underprivileged backgrounds in the preparation of their applications to study at large universities. This activity is based on crowdsourcing. Through an open call, Project Access encourages participants to provide related advice. The platform has managed to attract more than 5,000 collaborators and 3,300 applicants to universities since its foundation. Its model is similar to that implemented by CTI. Tutoring is performed individually and through digital media.

OPEN RESOURCES

In this case, open resources do not refer to the scientific texts on coronavirus discussed previously. Rather, they represent the materials that are available on the CTI website. This is a repository of resources that facilitate the preparation of the tutorials by volunteers. In addition, the participants have created a Facebook community in which they share tips and resources (Robertson, 2020). These resources facilitate the execution of the work. The tutors can raise any doubts they may have through this social network or consult the texts collected in the CTI repository. Thus, they can carry out their tasks properly.

NO ECONOMIC BENEFIT FOR THE CROWDSOURCER

CTI claims to be a nonprofit project. Its organizers do not benefit from the work done by its volunteers in an altruistic way. However, developing it has an economic cost. Therefore, it encourages people to make donations through its crowdfunding campaign, since they need financial aid to continue providing a free service to students who need it.

4.3.2.3 Barriers

NO TIME FOR PLANNING

Following the announcement of the closure of educational centers in the United Kingdom, one of the three university-aged organizers of CTI detected the impact that this would have on those schoolchildren whose families cannot afford private classes. He decided to help these students through free tutoring, and he sought the support of other university students to carry out this work. To do this, he posted a form on Facebook where interested parties could sign up. His idea was to manually connect volunteers and students. He did not have in mind creating a large crowd-sourcing project. However, he received more than 1,000 applications in 24 hours, and with the help of his colleagues, CTI was born (Tirahan, 2020).

DIGITAL DIVIDE

CTI acts to mitigate the effects that coronavirus can have on students from less privileged families. These students the ones who are the most vulnerable to the digital divide and may not have a device that allows them to access the platform on which the tutoring takes place. For this reason, the terms specify that students can request that the tutorials be carried out through other means if there is a lack of resources. This speci-fication is essential for all students to be able to receive the benefits of this project. Some households do not have devices with Internet access available for use by schoolchildren. In other households, the Internet connection is not adequate to use this service. Thinking about these and other assumptions, CTI aims to use alternative means to the Internet when necessary.

CYBERATTACKS

No reference has been made to an attack directed at this particular project or the platforms on which it is being developed at this time. However, it should be noted that there has been an increase in threats made to video conferencing applications, mainly Zoom. These applications have been widely used for work meetings and remote classes. The increase in the number of threats made regarding these applications is such that institu-tions such as the FBI have warned publicly about the presence of these threats and provided a series of tips to avoid being the victim of an attack, such as not making calls with free access and not publicly sharing the video conference link (FBI, 2020).

SENSITIVE DATA

The participants and students who request help through CTI must pro-vide their details, which allows them to be identified. In addition, the students are minors, so even more care must be taken to ensure that they will not be harmed. Therefore, CTI has developed a vast set of measures for their protection. These measures are included in a series of documents that can be freely accessed from the platform's website. In addition, they have created a team of volunteers who are responsible for ensuring the security of the project and safeguarding privacy. For example, sessions are recorded through the Bramble platform in case they need to be reviewed later by the CTI surveillance team.

DUPLICATED TASKS

No similar projects have been found to be developed within the same territory.

4.4 Other areas

4.4.1 Applications

The three applications mentioned previously are not the only ones in which crowdsourcing has been applied during this period; projects have also been created in other fields. One case is described below.

4.4.2 Case study: COVID Translate Project

The COVID Translate Project[11] is a crowdsourcing activity created by Sebastian Seung on March 27, 2020, to translate a Korean coronavirus action manual into English. To publicize the call, Seung used the social network platform of Twitter. The publication itself included a link to Google Docs to allow access to any individual who wanted to participate by editing the document. In just a few hours, he managed to recruit more than 50 volunteers. In two days, a preliminary version of the translated manuscript was achieved. On April 6, 2020, the work was completed, and the manuscript and its appendices were published in English. After that, other important texts concerning protocols and guidelines for action against COVID-19 continued to be translated. Other languages, such as Spanish, Italian, and Russian, have also been included.

4.4.2.1 Crowdsourcing elements

CROWDSOURCER

The crowdsourcer of the COVID Translate Project is Sebastian Seung, who is a professor at Princeton University (USA) and President of Samsung Research (Seung, 2020). Of Korean origin, Seung is aware of the quality of the action protocols against epidemics in this country as a consequence of the previous coronavirus that spread through it. For this reason, he detected the need to translate these guidelines into other languages to make them easier to read for the authorities responsible for managing this health crisis in other territories and, in this way, help to develop more effective measures. To achieve this, he decided to create the COVID Translate Project.

PLATFORM

Seung used his personal Twitter profile to launch the call. In a post on this social network, he explained the problem to his followers and asked for their help in carrying out the translation in a collaborative manner. He added a link to a Google Doc containing the text to be translated from Korean to English. Such Google Docs can be modified by any user who has permission to do so. Since this was crowdsourcing and the call was addressed to the entire population, the editing permission was open to any individual who wanted to access it. Later, a specific website for the project and profiles on Twitter and Facebook were created to publicize the results.

TASK

The task was to translate the Korean protocol provided by Seung into English. This was a complex task that required time to complete. Its execution was collaborative. All the participants had to translate the same text within the same document. Instead of dividing the text into smaller fragments, it was decided to create a single document and have it modified simultaneously by several people.

PARTICIPANTS

Participation is open to everyone. However, one has to have the capacity to be able to carry out the requested work. In particular, initially, it was necessary to know both Korean and English to translate the text from one language to the other. This was an informal requirement. In other words, the participants were not checked to see if they had this knowledge. Moreover, the language requirements for this platform are very specific. Therefore, the crowd to which the calls are addressed are not very large. Additionally, the participants are free to decide when to participate, for how many times and for how long. Anyone can access the texts at any time and spend either minutes or hours on the job, depending on their willingness.

4.4.2.2 Favorable conditions

MOTIVATED PARTICIPANTS

It can be said that the individuals who have collaborated in this project have done so altruistically to dedicate their efforts to help stop the spread of the virus. The dissemination of effective protocols against the virus facilitates decision-making regarding concerning the pandemic. This acts as a motivating element for the participants. Moreover, according to the crowdsourcer, participants believe in the cause (Seung, 2020). The call does not explicitly offer incentives but is a rather call for citizen collaboration. The volunteers do not receive any financial reward in return for their work. However, the COVID Translate Project's website displays the names of the nearly 200 volunteers, which provides a mechanism for recognition.

TIME TO PARTICIPATE

The tasks proposed by the COVID Translate Project require much time to be carried out. Translating is not a routine and simple activity. An effort must be made. Moreover, the technical language of the text in question increases its difficulty level since all individuals who know the Korean and English languages are not familiar with these technical elements. Therefore, this project benefits from the increased free time derived from confinement as volunteers can dedicate more minutes or hours to the task. However, it should be noted that the participants decide how much time they spend on it. This work is done jointly. An individual does not have to go to a certain extent for his or her task to be completed. That is, a user can stop his or her collaboration, and the activity will continue with other participants being able to continue where he or she has stopped the translation.

EASE OF DISSEMINATION

Seung spread the call through a publication on his personal Twitter account, which has 14,500 followers. This publication was shared by 1,300 users on this social network and obtained 2,400 likes. In other words, it had a direct impact on thousands of people. However, to participate in the initial call, one had to have a certain skill, namely, be able to translate from Korean to English. Therefore, participants not only needed the willingness to collaborate but also the ability to do so. Despite this barrier, more than 50 people started editing the document in the first few hours. According to their website, almost 200 participated throughout the activity.

CROWDSOURCER'S EXPERIENCE

The success of this project is not due to luck. Seung is a professor at Princeton University and has experience in the field of crowdsourcing. He leads the Eyewire project,[12] which is a game launched in 2012 that aims to map the structure of neurons. This crowdsourcing activity is based on citizen science. It proposes that participants solve puzzles. Its resolutions are the contributions received by the organizer. Thanks to these contributions, scientific advances have been published in various journals.

In the face of the COVID-19 crisis, Seung used his knowledge of the field to obtain the translation of a Korean protocol manual thanks to the collaboration of citizens. He then offered a series of recommendations via Twitter to ensure the success of future crowdsourcing calls (Seung, 2020). These recommendations are as follows:

(1) Explain significance. His Twitter appeal said "SAVE LIVES by translating Korean -> English!," which summarize the purpose of the call.
(2) Set a deadline. The crowd was asked to participate by the Monday following the post. Seung says that deadlines evoke a sense of urgency that causes the public to act more quickly.
(3) Quantify progress. The goal was to translate 75 pages. This numerical quantification allows users to know what percentage of the task has been carried out and how much is left to finish.
(4) Make an open call. Despite the difficulty involved in a complex task such as translating a technical document, Seung chose to allow the participation of any individual. He argues that projects often require diverse skills and experience levels.
(5) Facilitate immediate participation. The publication on Twitter that included the announcement incorporated the Google Docs link that provided access the document. Seung argues that he considered the option of having the public send an email to request permission, but this would cause delays in the process and demotivate participants.
(6) Trust strangers. Open access to a document generates vulnerability to attacks. However, Google Docs allows you to go back and undo changes. This eliminates the potential problem of vulnerability. In addition, Seung emphasizes the low probability of this happening.
(7) Make it social. The crowdsourcer of this project maintains that volunteers initially participate for the cause but that they remain because

of the bonds they create with the community. Therefore, interaction between the participants should be encouraged. In Google Docs, this is done through comments, internal chats, and the visualization of the users who are connected at that moment.

(8)   Attract an audience. Seung claims that it is not only the participants who are part of the project but also other Internet users who, although not participating, follow the development of the call and are thus also part of it and encourage those who contribute.

(9)   Quality control. Establish quality standards and monitor the participants' compliance.

(10) Show results early and recurrent. The first versions of the translated text were published without being completely accurate. However, institutions could already start to benefit from their use and adapt their measures to these protocols.

(11) Disseminate the results. To generate impact, the results must be publicized. Seung chose to create the project's website and profiles on Twitter and Facebook and spread them from those points.

(12) Analyze website traffic. With the benefit of such analysis, it can be known what kind of impact the project is having.

(13) Do not be discouraged by the detractors. This call received various criticisms. Among them was the possibility of obtaining an inaccurate translation by carrying out such a service through crowdsourcing.

(14) Have fun.

OPEN RESOURCES

In this case, the protocol to be translated was provided by the crowdsourcer. The participants did not have to do any search work. They only had to use their knowledge of both languages to achieve the objective of the call.

NO ECONOMIC BENEFIT FOR THE CROWDSOURCER

The COVID Translate Project is not for profit. Its aim is to translate effective action protocols to help stop the coronavirus as quickly as possible. This is intended to help governments of other countries deal with the pandemic. The translated documents are made public. Any individual or entity can access them via the Internet. The results of this project help to improve the global knowledge about coronavirus and the measures that can be applied to stop its expansion, without its organizer obtaining any economic benefit in return.

4.4.2.3 Barriers

NO TIME FOR PLANNING

No data have been found about the time that passed from the time the crowdsourcer decided to create the project until the time when it was launched. However, this time was surely brief. No specific platform was created, but a Google Doc was used that could be freely modified. The description of the call was made through a thread of publications on Twitter, with the first publication providing the essential information. The rest was used to justify the need for collaboration.

Since Seung has experience with crowdsourcing, one can say that he applied his knowledge of the field to develop an effective project as quickly as possible. To do so, he opted to use existing platforms that did not need any adaptation to host the call. This made it easier to reduce the planning and design time.

DIGITAL DIVIDE

Only those individuals with an Internet connection can access this call. Therefore, it is affected by the digital divide, since there is a group of the population that cannot collaborate in the activity. Even so, the purpose of the project is to provide resources to governments to facilitate decision-making regarding measures to help control the epidemic. If these measures are developed, they will be implemented throughout an entire territory, thereby affecting the population as a whole. All citizens will benefit from their effects regardless of whether they have been able to participate in it or not. The digital divide only affects the possibility of collaboration. However, it does not distinguish between who takes advantage of the results since these take place outside the digital sphere.

CYBERATTACKS

The COVID Translate Project is a particularly vulnerable activity. Participation takes place through a document that can be modified by anyone. There is no mechanism to control who accesses the document or the quality of the contributions. It is possible for an individual to behave dishonestly and act against the call. It is not necessary to have computer skills to attack the project and damage the results. Even so, there is no record of anyone acting against it. The crowdsourcer was aware of this threat but decided to use this tool to host the activity. An open document speeds up the process as it involves fewer technical requirements. For example, the participants do not have to spend time on registration and can thus spend all their efforts on translation. In addition, Google Docs allow users to undo changes. If an attack occurs, the text can be restored to its previous state. In addition, the crowdsourcer emphasizes that people should be trusted. The project has a goal that benefits society as a whole. Therefore, Seung argues that such attacks are unlikely to happen (Seung, 2020).

SENSITIVE DATA

No registration of volunteers is required to participate. Therefore, they do not provide any sensitive data.

DUPLICATED TASKS

No similar project has been created. That is, this is the only one that has presented a task with these characteristics.

Notes

1 www.frenalacurva.net
2 www.covidibd.org
3 www.covidceliac.org
4 www.rheum-covd.org
5 https://covid.joinzoe.com
6 https://covid19.nhs.uk/
7 www.coronavirustutoring.co.uk
8 www.projectaccess.org
9 www.bramble.io
10 www.getadapt.co.uk
11 www.covidtranslate.org
12 www.eyewire.org

Bibliographic references

Agerholm, H. (2020, May 23). Coronavirus: Five things a Covid-19 symptom-tracking app tells us. *BBC*. Retrieved September 16, 2020, from https://www.bbc.com/news/health-52770313

Ahn, J. M., Roijakkers, N., Fini, R., & Mortara, L. (2019). Leveraging open innovation to improve society: Past achievements and future trajectories. *R&D Management, 49*(3), 267–278.

Coronavirus Tutoring Initiative [@CoronaTutoring]. (2020a, April 30). *Jess says' I signed up tutor with @CoronaTutoring because I wanted to do something worthwhile and to give back! I* [Tweet]. Retrieved July 17, 2020, from https://twitter.com/CoronaTutoring/status/1255841648434708482

Coronavirus Tutoring Initiative [@CoronaTutoring]. (2020b, May 4). *I joined the initiatve because I don't think that children should lose out on education as a result of the* [Tweet]. Retrieved July 17, 2020, from https://twitter.com/CoronaTutoring/status/1257326688045801474

Coronavirus Tutoring Initiative [@CoronaTutoring]. (2020c, May 9). *The project is a great idea to keep a relaxed academic vibe present in student's lives to try keep some* [Tweet]. Retrieved July 17, 2020, from https://twitter.com/CoronaTutoring/status/1259140608523939841

Coronavirus Tutoring Initiative [@CoronaTutoring]. (2020d, April 21). *Teachers and parents- we would be very grateful if you could RETWEET this and pass on the message to any* [Tweet]. Retrieved July 17, 2020, from https://twitter.com/CoronaTutoring/status/1252553742785929222

Covid19People. (2020). *Municipal chamber of Câmara de Lobos.* Retrieved September 1, 2020, from https://pt.covid19people.help/issues/41/

Davis, N. (2020, March 24). UK app aims to help researchers track spread of coronavirus. *The Guardian.* Retrieved September 16, 2020, from https://www.theguardian.com/science/2020/mar/24/uk-app-aims-to-help-researchers-track-spread-of-coronavirus

Elcheroth, G., & Drury, J. (2020). Collective resilience in times of crisis: Lessons from the literature for socially effective responses to the pandemic. *British Journal of Social Psychology, 59*(3), 703–713.

FBI. (2020, March 30). *FBI warns of teleconferencing and online classroom hijacking during COVID-19 pandemic.* Retrieved September 20, 2020, from https://www.fbi.gov/contact-us/field-offices/boston/news/press-releases/fbi-warns-of-teleconferencing-and-online-classroom-hijacking-during-covid-19-pandemic

Freeman, E. E., McMahon, D. E., Fitzgerald, M. E., Fox, L. P., Rosenbach, M., Takeshita, J., . . . Hruza, G. J. (2020). The American academy of dermatology COVID-19 registry: Crowdsourcing dermatology in the age of COVID-19. *Journal of the American Academy of Dermatology, 83*(2), 509–510.

Frena La Curva [@frenalacurva]. (2020a, June 22). *Y llegamos a la #NuevaNormalidad Nunca olvidaremos el gran esfuerzo que hemos hecho tod@s para #frenarlacurva y llegar hasta la* [Tweet]. Retrieved September 14, 2020, from https://twitter.com/frenalacurva/status/1275004436629401600

Frena La Curva. (2020b). *Clipping FLC.* Retrieved September 14, 2020, from https://docs.google.com/spreadsheets/d/1DTsugDFwQs6DTOIU6gHGqfkykvRkXOQFN7UmJRmEfBk/edit?usp=sharing

Frena La Curva. (2020c). *Qué es FLC.* Retrieved September 15, 2020, from https://frenalacurva.net/conocenos-frena-la-curva

Fuger, S., Schimpf, R., Füller, J., & Hutter, K. (2017). User roles and team structures in a crowdsourcing community for international development-a social network perspective. *Information Technology for Development, 23*(3), 438–462.

Hosseini, M., Angelopoulos, C. M., Chai, W. K., & Kundig, S. (2019). Crowdcloud: A crowdsourced system for cloud infrastructure. *Cluster Computing, 22*(2), 455–470.

Impact Hub. (n.d.). *Quiénes somos.* Retrieved September 20, 2020, from https://madrid.impacthub.net/quienes-somos/

Instituto de Estudios Económicos Provincia de Alicante. (2020, April 27). *#tomamitablet #tomamiportatil.* Retrieved September 4, 2020, from https://ineca-alicante.es/noticias/tomamitablet-tomamiportatil/

Jacobs, A. (2020, May 11). App shows promise in tracking new Coronavirus cases, study finds. *The New York Times*. Retrieved September 9, 2020, from https://www.nytimes.com/2020/05/11/health/coronavirus-symptoms-app.html

Kaleidos. (2020a, March 20). *Un mapa colaborativo de ayuda vecinal para "frenar la curva"*. Retrieved September 20, 2020, from https://blog.kaleidos.net/mapa-colaborativo-ayuda-voluntariado-vecinal-coronavirus/

Kaleidos. (2020b, April 7). *Frena La Curva Maps, conectando hispano-hablantes con recursos críticos en su entorno*. Retrieved September 20, 2020, from https://blog.kaleidos.net/frenalacurvamaps-conectado-hispanohablantes-recursos-criticos-con-ushahidi/

Laboratorio de Aragón Gobierno Abierto [LAAAB]. (2020, March 18). Trabajamos para frenar la curva [Blog post]. *Blog Laboratorio de Aragón Gobierno Abierto*. Retrieved August 25, 2020, from http://www.laaab.es/2020/03/trabajamos-para-frenar-la-curva/

Leung, G. M., & Leung, K. (2020). Crowdsourcing data to mitigate epidemics. *The Lancet Digital Health, 2*(4), e156–e157.

Liu, A., Wang, W., Shang, S., Li, Q., & Zhang, X. (2018). Efficient task assignment in spatial crowdsourcing with worker and task privacy protection. *GeoInformatica, 22*(2), 335–362.

Misra, R. (2020, March 15). 5 ways to help your community combat Coronavirus (while still social distancing). *The New York Times*. Retrieved October 12, 2020, from https://www.nytimes.com/2020/03/15/smarter-living/wirecutter/5-ways-to-help-during-coronavirus-while-social-distancing.html

Mulenga, E. M., & Marbán, J. M. (2020). Is COVID-19 the gateway for digital learning in mathematics education? *Contemporary Educational Technology, 12*(2), ep269.

Robertson, X. (2020). "Coronavirus tutoring project": How one Oxford student is helping thousands of children in lockdown. *The Cambridge Tab*. Retrieved September 17, 2020, from https://thetab.com/uk/cambridge/2020/06/12/coronavirus-tutoring-project-how-one-oxford-student-is-helping-thousands-of-children-in-lockdown-138792

Robinson, P. C., & Yazdany, J. (2020). The COVID-19 global rheumatology alliance: Collecting data in a pandemic. *Nature Reviews Rheumatology, 16*, 293–294.

Seung, S. [@SebastianSeung]. (2020, March 31). Crowdsourcing *can indeed be powerful. 75 pages translated last weekend, lightning speed for a complex technical document. I believe that* [Tweet thread]. Twitter. Retrieved September 14, 2020, from https://twitter.com/SebastianSeung/status/1245012707549548544

Spector, T., & Chan, A. (2020, May 11). Coronavirus: Research reveals way to predict infection - without a test. *The Conversation*. Retrieved September 15, 2020, from https://theconversation.com/coronavirus-research-reveals-way-to-predict-infection-without-a-test-138284.

Tirahan, L. (2020, April 16). Jacob Kelly: Founder of the tutoring project promoting free education amid school closures. *The Oxford Student*. Retrieved September 20, 2020, from https://www.oxfordstudent.com/2020/04/16/jacob-kelly-founder-of-the-tutoring-project-promoting-free-education-amid-school-closures/

TwinsUK. (2020a). *About us*. Retrieved September 15, 2020, from https://twinsuk.ac.uk/about-us/what-is-twinsuk

TwinsUK. (2020b, March 20). *TwinsUK to start COVID-19 research*. Retrieved September 15, 2020, from https://twinsuk.ac.uk/twinsuk-to-start-covid-19-research/

UNESCO. (2020). *COVID-19 impact on education.* Retrieved September 5, 2020, from https://en.unesco.org/covid19/educationresponse

Volpicelli, G. (2020, March 26). The inside story of the UK's biggest coronavirus symptom tracker app. *Wired.* Retrieved September 16, 2020, from https://www.wired.co.uk/article/covid-symptom-tracker-app-coronavirus-uk

ZOE. (2020a, August 18). *Department of health issues grant to COVID symptom study.* COVID Symptom Study-Join ZOE. Retrieved September 16, 2020, from https://covid.joinzoe.com/post/grant

ZOE. (2020b, March 26). *Over 1 million citizen scientists and counting!* COVID Symptom Study- Join ZOE. Retrieved September 16, 2020, from https://covid.joinzoe.com/post/over-1-million-citizen-scientists-and-counting

ZOE. (2020c, April 11). *First minister mark drakefors makes urgent appeal.* COVID Symptom Study- Join ZOE. Retrieved September 16, 2020, from https://covid.joinzoe.com/post/nhs-wales.

ZOE. (2020d, March 30). *Webinar: Symptom analysis.* COVID Symptom Study- Join ZOE. Retrieved September 16, 2020, from https://covid.joinzoe.com/post/covid-research-update-uk

ZOE. (2020e, March 29). *Join our COVID-19 webinar tomorrow to hear what leading scientists have learned from our COVID symptom tracker app. register here.* COVID Symptom Study- Join ZOE [Facebook Post]. Retrieved September 16, 2020, from https://m.facebook.com/joinzoe1/photos/a.477253323050165/686792788762883/?type=3&source=57&__tn__=EH-R

ZOE. (2020f). *About us.* COVID Symptom Study- Join ZOE. Retrieved September 27, 2020, from https://joinzoe.com/about-zoe

5 Conclusions and final reflections

The new coronavirus has caused an unprecedented crisis worldwide. Exceptional measures have been taken to stop its expansion, and research has been accelerated to determine how it behaves and, relatedly, to find effective strategies to combat it. In this context, where social distancing is required and the majority of the population is confined to their homes, crowdsourcing has been very useful. In this book, we have explained how this tool has been used, and we have examined a series of factors that have facilitated and hindered the development of these projects. Specifically, Chapter 3 discusses various favorable conditions and barriers that have affected crowdsourcing during this pandemic period. These factors are analyzed through the study of four cases in the following fourth chapter. The following conclusions can be drawn from this analysis.

First, these cases exemplify the plurality of applications and features that crowdsourcing can present. Regarding the purpose of these projects, they have been used, on the one hand, to advance the research and dissemination of knowledge about the coronavirus. In the healthcare field, an application has been created that, thanks to the monitoring of numerous individuals, has made it possible to improve the understanding of the symptoms and behavior of the coronavirus disease. Crowdsourcing has also enabled the spread of useful information through the collaborative translation of protocols of action against coronavirus.

On the other hand, projects have been designed to help the most vulnerable populations. At the educational level, they have been developed to help students who are members of families with fewer resources. At the social levels, they have been developed to help individuals who need support to carry out daily activities. These cases also illustrate the variety of profiles that can act as crowdsourcers: individuals, associations of citizens, entities, and institutions of various kinds. In addition, the multiple levels of complexity of the task requested from the crowd have been

DOI: 10.4324/9781003290872-5

highlighted, from spending one minute a day reporting individual symptoms to spending several hours offering tutorials or translating texts.

Special mention should be made of the platforms that have been used in this context. Specific websites and applications have been developed for Frena La Curva and the COVID Symptom Study. The first website is based on technology available from Ushahidi, a recurrent platform for crisis management through crowdsourcing. The second website is without a previously existing base. On the other hand, CTI and the COVID Translate Project, although they have web pages detailing the terms of both calls, do not take place on crowdsourcing platforms.

CTI tutoring is offered through Bramble, an existing digital platform that connects tutors and students. The translation of the COVID Translate Project has been executed in a Google Docs–based collaborative editing document. This highlights the possibility of leveraging resources that, although not designed for crowdsourcing, can be adapted and used as a basis for these activities to take place. That is, it is not necessary to create a platform to launch a call or to resort to open platforms that provide this service to multiple crowdsourcers in exchange for a fee.

From the analysis of the factors that may have helped crowdsourcing during this period in the four exposed cases, several conclusions can be drawn. The first is the motivation of the participants to participate in these projects. During the beginning of the pandemic, there were calls for selfless collaboration to address the crisis and mitigate its effects. The four examples discussed in this paper share a common motivation: altruism. Studies support the idea that this factor acts as an incentive in crowdsourcing (Alam et al., 2020; Cappa et al., 2019b; Schäper et al., 2020). Moreover, none of them offer remuneration for participation. All of them rely on the willingness to help others, either directly, such as Frena La Curva and CTI, or indirectly, such as the COVID Symptom Study and the COVID Translate Project, which are aimed at research and policy development. This reliance is related to another favorable factor, namely, the absence of economic benefit for the crowdsourcer. They are nonprofit, and their results will not be commercialized. Both factors seem to have motivating elements that have contributed to crowdsourcing during this pandemic period.

Another reason is the increase in free time. In the case of tasks that require more dedication, such as CTI tutoring or the translation involved in the COVID Translate Project, this factor could be key to their success. Regarding their dissemination, all of the projects use social networks. Basing their communication strategy on social network channels does not entail any cost. It is a fast and effective option that constitutes an alternative to accessing the knowledge and experience of the crowd

(Candi et al., 2018). This aspect has been enhanced by the increased time spent on these media during the home confinement (Cellini et al., 2020; Rodriguez-Rey et al., 2020; Sinha et al., 2020). A clear example of this is the COVID Translate Project. Its crowdsourcer used only his Twitter profile, which has a large number of followers, to publicize the activity. With this post, the crowdsourcer managed to reach a sufficient number of individuals to achieve his goal in a few days. In addition, some of the calls analyzed herein have benefited from their appearance in the media. This appearance increases the number of potential participants. On the other hand, it should be noted that the existence of open resources, which has been identified as one of the possible facilitating factors of crowdsourcing, has not had any effect on the cases described.

The last favorable factor is the experience of the crowdsourcer. The organizers of the four cases have previously carried out crowdsourcing and open innovation projects or have allied with agents who have done so. This may be a reason why the possible barrier of having little time to plan has not affected them negatively. The crowdsourcers acted quickly by detecting needs and designing calls to solve them through citizen collaboration. Experience is a factor that facilitates crowdsourcing (Blohm et al., 2018; Thuan et al., 2016). It can be argued that creating other calls has helped reduce the time needed to design these calls during the onset of the pandemic and that these calls have been successfully developed.

Another possible obstacle refers to the increase in cyberattacks during this pandemic period (INTERPOL, 2020). However, there is no evidence that such attacks have been directed at the cases examined. Similarly, requiring the contribution of sensitive data can discourage participation in crowdsourcing (Alorwu et al., 2020). To address this issue, the projects analyzed herein have sought to ensure the privacy of their users by avoiding requesting information that allows users to be identified, for example, by eliminating the need to register in order to contribute or by asking for as little information as possible. In the event that the collection of such information is essential to carrying out the work, as in the case of CTI, the platforms have created a team to ensure the security of the agents involved in the activity.

Since crowdsourcing takes place over the Internet, the digital divide can negatively affect the subsets of the population that do not have the capacity to operate in this environment. This is especially important when activities are intended to help the most vulnerable individuals, as both groups may overlap (Beaunoyer et al., 2020). To address this issue, the above calls have resorted to different strategies, such as allowing a third-party agent to participate on behalf of a subject. In this way, the number of participants is increased, thereby mitigating the effects of the digital divide and achieving a greater volume of contributions. The duplication of tasks in more than one crowdsourcing activity did not have a negative influence on the cases analyzed.

Finally, it is worth noting a phenomenon that has occurred in three of the cases analyzed, namely, the increase in their scope. This phenomenon consists of adding more population groups to those targeted by the call. Frena La Curva, after its start in Spain, has been replicated in more than 20 countries. These are projects with the same name that are managed by different crowdsourcers. The COVID Symptom Study originated in the United Kingdom and was later launched in the United States and Sweden. For this purpose, its original organizers joined forces with researchers from these territories. The third case is the COVID Translate Project. At first, this call requested the translation of a text from Korean to English. After that, the population was urged to translate the protocol into other languages. In this way, the call was directed to other individuals who, although they did not have the skills to collaborate in the first activity, could intervene in subsequent calls.

The lessons gleaned herein regarding the fight against coronavirus through crowdsourcing can be applied in future projects. In particular, lessons regarding how they have taken advantage of different factors that act in their favor and how they have solved other issues that worked against them will be useful in the future. This knowledge can be used to develop other calls, regardless of whether they are enacted in a moment of crisis or not, thereby enabling them to be carried out successfully. Likewise, future lines of research should be aimed at deepening the knowledge about these features and identifying other factors that also affect crowdsourcing. Furthermore, it is advisable to engage in future studies of the effects of these factors in a quantitative way to develop guidelines that help to improve the effectiveness of these activities and help participants make decisions regarding their design.

Bibliographic references

Alam, S. L., Sun, R., & Campbell, J. (2020). Helping yourself or others? Motivation dynamics for high-performing volunteers in GLAM crowdsourcing. *Australasian Journal of Information Systems, 24.*

Alorwu, A., van Berkel, N., Goncalves, J., Oppenlaender, J., López, M. B., Seetharaman, M., & Hosio, S. (2020). Crowdsourcing sensitive data using public displays-opportunities, challenges, and considerations. *Personal and Ubiquitous Computing.* https://doi.org/10.1007/s00779-020-01375-6.

Beaunoyer, E., Dupéré, S., & Guitton, M. J. (2020). COVID-19 and digital inequalities: Reciprocal impacts and mitigation strategies. *Computers in Human Behavior, 111,* 106424.

Blohm, I., Zogaj, S., Bretschneider, U., & Leimeister, J. M. (2018). How to manage crowdsourcing platforms effectively? *California Management Review, 60*(2), 122–149.

Candi, M., Roberts, D. L., Marion, T., & Barczak, G. (2018). Social strategy to gain knowledge for innovation. *British Journal of Management, 29*(4), 731–749.

Cappa, F., Rosso, F., & Hayes, D. (2019). Monetary and social rewards for crowdsourcing. *Sustainability, 11*(10), 2834.

Cellini, N., Canale, N., Mioni, G., & Costa, S. (2020). Changes in sleep pattern, sense of time and digital media use during COVID-19 lockdown in Italy. *Journal of Sleep Research*, e13074.

INTERPOL. (2020, August). *COVID-19 cybercrime analysis report*. Retrieved September 4, 2020, from https://www.interpol.int/News-and-Events/News/2020/INTERPOL-report-shows-alarming-rate-of-cyberattacks-during-COVID-19

Rodríguez-Rey, R., Garrido-Hernansaiz, H., & Collado, S. (2020). Psychological impact and associated factors during the initial stage of the coronavirus (COVID-19) pandemic among the general population in Spain. *Frontiers in Psychology, 11*, 1540.

Schäper, T., Foege, J. N., Nüesch, S., & Schäfer, S. (2020). Determinants of idea sharing in crowdsourcing: Evidence from the automotive industry. *R&D Management, 51*(1), 101–113.

Sinha, M., Pande, B., & Sinha, R. (2020). Impact of COVID-19 lockdown on sleep-wake schedule and associated lifestyle related behavior: A national survey. *Journal of Public Health Research, 9*(3).

Thuan, N. H., Antunes, P., & Johnstone, D. (2016). Factors influencing the decision to crowdsource: A systematic literature review. *Information Systems Frontiers, 18*(1), 47–68.

Index